Practical Psychology

for
DIABETES CLINICIANS

2ND EDITION

Barbara J. Anderson, PhD, and
Richard R. Rubin, PhD, CDE, Editors

American Diabetes Association.

*Cure • Care • Commitment*SM

Director, Book Publishing, John Fedor; Associate Director, Professional Books, Christine B. Welch; Editor, Joyce Raynor; Project Manager/Editor, Wendy Martin; Production Manager, Peggy M. Rote; Composition, Circle Graphics, Inc.; Cover Design, SueEllen Lawton; Printer, Hamilton Printing Co.

Printed in the United States of America
1 3 5 7 9 10 8 6 4 2

ADA titles may be purchased for business or promotional use or for special sales. For information, please write to Lee Romano Sequeira, Special Sales & Promotions, at the address below or at LRomano@diabetes.org or call 703-299-2046.

American Diabetes Association
1701 North Beauregard Street
Alexandria, Virginia 22311

Library of Congress Cataloging-in-Publication Data
Practical psychology for diabetes clinicians / Barbara J. Anderson, Richard R. Rubin, editors.— 2nd ed.
    p. ; cm.
    Includes bibliographical references and index.
    ISBN 1-58040-140-6 (pbk. : alk. paper)
    1. Diabetes—Psychological aspects. 2. Clinical health psychology. I. Anderson, Barbara J. (Barbara Jane), 1947- II. Rubin, Richard R. III. American Diabetes Association.
    [DNLM: 1. Diabetes Mellitus—psychology. 2. Diabetes Mellitus—therapy. WK 810 P895 2002]
RC660 .P725 2002
616.4'62'0019—dc21   2002066621

Contents

II

III

IV

*Understanding Psychological Issues
That Affect Self-Care*   209

AFTERWORD

INDEX

Preface

Diabetes treatment today is a good news–bad news story. The good news is abundant: we have new tools for monitoring and controlling blood glucose levels and other risk factors for complications. Unfortunately, the bad news is also plentiful: type 2 diabetes is an epidemic throughout the world, fueled substantially by changes in lifestyle and now affecting children as well as adults. In addition, most people who have diabetes are not realistically able to take full advantage of the tools available for managing their disease; as a result, many continue to suffer from chronically high blood glucose levels and long-term diabetes complications.

This gap between the potential of diabetes treatment and its actual accomplishments emphasizes the critical role of self-care in determining diabetes outcomes. The past 20 years have seen a dramatic increase in the volume and quality of behavioral research in diabetes, focused on efforts to understand and facilitate self-care.

The Council on Behavioral Medicine and Psychology of the American Diabetes Association developed the first edition of this book in 1996 to provide diabetes clinicians with the latest behavioral information on diabetes management. We asked leading behavioral science researchers in diabetes to translate their findings into guidelines for physicians, nurses, dietitians, exercise physiologists, and mental health professionals who care for people with diabetes. This second edition of *Practical Psychology for Diabetes Clinicians* contains a wealth of information generated over the past 6 years, including new chapters on working with patient interpersonal interaction styles, tailoring care to minority patients and their families, using interactive technology to facilitate self-care, helping patients develop diabetes coping skills, working with young adults who have type 1 diabetes, identifying and treating youth who have type 2 diabetes, preventing type 2 diabetes in adults, and treating eating disorders in young women who have type 1 diabetes.

We divided the book into four parts. The first includes chapters on interacting effectively with patients. The second part contains chapters on facilitating diabetes self-care behaviors. The third part offers guidelines for responding to developmental and family influences on self-care, and the last part is designed to help clinicians understand psychological issues that affect diabetes self-care.

Each part offers guidance for diabetes clinicians dealing with a wide range of concerns, from tailoring care to minority patients, to helping patients increase their activity levels, control their weight, or stop smoking, to recognizing the impact of depression in people with diabetes.

We hope this book gives you some practical recommendations for handling the critical behavioral issues you and your patients confront.

Barbara J. Anderson, PhD
Richard R. Rubin, PhD, CDE

PART One

Interacting Effectively with Patients

The vast majority of diabetes care is self-care. Countless times each day people with diabetes make choices that affect their health. Helping patients make these choices wisely is challenging because most clinicians were trained to deliver care and not to facilitate self-care. This challenge is often compounded by a lack of time in the clinical interaction and cultural differences between clinician and patient. The first part of this book addresses the importance of the patient-clinician relationship.

In the first chapter, R. Anderson and Funnell describe the empowerment approach to helping people change behavior. This approach is based on the reality that people change their behavior when (and only when) these changes are personally meaningful to them. Through a series of examples, the authors demonstrate an approach to helping patients make personally meaningful changes in diabetes self-care.

In his chapter, Ciechanowski points out that clinicians can improve interactions with patients and clinical outcomes when they are able to recognize and work with a patient's individual interpersonal style. The author offers a practical way to assess interpersonal styles, using the construct of attachment theory along with guidelines for responding effectively to various styles.

The clinician's emotional state can also powerfully affect interactions with patients. In her chapter, Hanson explains what happens when diabetes clinicians "burn out." She looks at some of the factors that contribute to diabetes clinician burnout and offers practical strategies for preventing and treating burnout.

The experience of having diabetes and caring for it can vary dramatically according to a person's race and ethnicity. In their chapter, Nwankwo and Tang offer guidelines for "walking into" the cultural lives and beliefs of minority patients, families, and communities. They show how this can help clinicians and patients form a more collaborative approach to diabetes care to help minority patients integrate diabetes care into their lives.

1

Using the Empowerment Approach to Help Patients Change Behavior

ROBERT M. ANDERSON, EdD,
AND MARTHA M. FUNNELL, MS, RN, CDE

This chapter describes the empowerment approach as a method for helping patients select and make changes in their diabetes self-management. This approach is based on principles of counseling and educational psychology, nursing and behavioral change theory, and the reality of day-to-day management of a chronic disease such as diabetes. The changing roles of health care providers and patients required by this approach are also discussed.

LEARN ABOUT THE PRINCIPLES OF EMPOWERMENT

The empowerment approach is based on three key principles related to diabetes, its management, and the psychology of behavior change. The principles are summarized below.

1. The reality of diabetes care is that more than 98% of that care is provided by the patient; therefore, the patient is the locus of control and decision-making in the daily treatment of diabetes.
2. The primary mission of the health care team is to provide ongoing diabetes expertise, education, and psychosocial support so that patients can make informed decisions about their daily diabetes self-management.

3. Adults are much more likely to make and maintain behavior changes if those changes are personally meaningful and freely chosen.

UNDERSTAND THE DIFFERENCE BETWEEN ACUTE DISEASE CARE AND CHRONIC DISEASE CARE

In the treatment of acute diseases, the health care professional is the primary decision-maker and is generally in control of treatment. The treatment of diabetes requires a different approach because it is a self-management disease. The health care professional has four major responsibilities to the patient in the treatment of diabetes:

1. Provide the diabetes expertise required for the development of an effective diabetes self-management plan.
2. Educate patients so that they can make informed decisions.
3. Create a collaborative relationship with patients and their families so that self-management plans can be reviewed and revised as necessary.
4. Provide the support necessary for patients to make and sustain self-selected behavior changes.

The behavior changes required for diabetes self-management need to be selected by the patient rather than imposed by the health care professional. This approach to diabetes care represents a significant change in the traditional relationship between patient and professional and requires new roles from both parties. Patients need to understand that the daily care of their diabetes is their personal responsibility. They are also responsible for establishing a partnership with their health care professionals. Health care professionals need to redefine their role as an advisor and collaborator and the patient's role as the decision-maker.

UNDERSTAND THE HEALTH CARE PROFESSIONAL'S CHALLENGES IN USING EMPOWERMENT

There are two major challenges health care professionals often face in successfully implementing the empowerment approach to diabetes care.

1. The first challenge is the discomfort some health care professionals experience when discussing the emotional content of diabetes

or a diabetes problem that a patient has identified. Having and caring for diabetes has a potent emotional component for most patients. Adults seldom make and sustain significant changes in their lives unless they feel a strong need to change. If the change process is to be successful, it is crucial for the health care professional to elicit the patient's feelings related to the issue. If the patient does not experience strong (usually negative) feelings about the current situation, the likelihood of sustained behavior change is small. Health care professionals are not required to solve or change patients' emotions (i.e., make them feel better) but rather to create an environment in which the patient's emotional experience is validated and can be expressed freely.

2. The second major challenge is the tendency of many health care professionals to solve problems for patients rather than with them. If a patient is clearly asking for technical expertise possessed by the health care professional, such behavior is appropriate. For example, if a patient says "I don't know how to make my glucose meter work," the appropriate response is to teach the patient the required technique. However, most of the problems involved in the daily treatment of diabetes are more psychosocial than technical, e.g., "I find it really difficult to cut back on fat when my family insists on fried foods all the time." The solution to the second kind of problem must come from the patient if it is to be implemented successfully. The process of helping patients discover their capacity to solve their own problems reinforces their self-efficacy and personal responsibility for the treatment of their diabetes.

UNDERSTAND PATIENT CHALLENGES TO USING EMPOWERMENT

There are also challenges that patients may need to face to successfully implement this approach to diabetes care. Many patients are so used to being blamed and criticized for their efforts at diabetes self-management that they are reluctant to visit health care professionals, discuss openly their daily efforts related to diabetes care, express any disagreement with a health care professional, and assert their own needs or values related to the treatment of their diabetes. All of the above actions are necessary to successfully manage diabetes. For health care professionals to use the empowerment approach successfully, their patients need to understand that they are equal partners in the care process.

KNOW HOW TO HELP PATIENTS WITH EMPOWERMENT

The following protocol is designed to help patients:

- Realize that they are responsible for and in charge of the daily treatment of their diabetes.
- Prioritize their diabetes-related problems and identify situations they want to improve.
- Experience the emotional and psychological commitment necessary to make and sustain a behavior change.
- Develop a behavior change plan.
- Evaluate their behavior change plan.

USE A BEHAVIOR CHANGE PROTOCOL

The following protocol is a series of questions to help patients identify and commit to a behavior change plan. The questions follow a logical sequence in terms of identifying problems, moving toward their solution, and evaluating the outcome. However, because empowerment is an overall approach to care and not a technique, we are *not* suggesting that the questions be used as a rigid sequence for interacting with patients. There are many situations in which the natural flow of the interaction would result in a discussion of the questions in a different order and/or the addition or deletion of some questions.

The protocol is meant to provide guidance in helping patients consider how they can make changes in their diabetes self-management. There may be instances when the health care professional will need to provide information about diabetes care during the discussion. With some patients, the behavior change plan may focus on short-term behavioral goals so that patients can experience the change process and become familiar with an incremental approach to behavior change. With other patients, the focus may be on the acquisition of the information and skills necessary to make informed choices. These questions are meant to help support a process of patient-centered decision-making. No matter how much or how little patients know about diabetes, they are capable of making changes as long as they have some insight into their own behavior. This protocol is equally effective in an individual or group situation. In a group situation, you can ask patients to write down each question. You can also consider asking participants to volunteer a problem or to work one-on-one with the educator in front of the group.

What part of living with diabetes is most difficult or unsatisfying? (Would you tell me more about that? Would you give me some specific examples? Would you paint a picture of the situation for me?)

The purpose of this question is to focus the discussion on the patient's concerns about living with and caring for diabetes. Clinicians and patients often have different priorities about the most important issues related to diabetes care. Patients are most likely to make changes that will solve problems that are personally meaningful and relevant to them.

How does that (the situation described above) make you feel? (Are you feeling [insert the feeling, e.g., angry, sad, confused, etc.]? Are you feeling [insert the feeling] because [insert the reason]?)

As mentioned earlier, patients seldom make and sustain changes in situations unless they care deeply about solving the problem or improving the situation. It is common for people to repress uncomfortable emotions, and repressed emotions reduce the energy and clarity necessary for effective problem-solving (see Chapter 20).

Discussing the feelings associated with a particular diabetes care situation can energize patients. When patients experience the depth of their anger, sadness, or dissatisfaction by talking about their feelings, they are much more likely to take action.

How would this situation have to change for you to feel better about it? (Where would you like to be regarding this situation in [insert specific time, e.g., 1 month, 3 months]? What will happen if you don't do anything to change this situation? How will you feel if things don't change?)

The purpose of this question is to help patients identify concretely how the situation would appear if it were improved. This means imagining the particulars of the situation if it were to be changed and imagining how they would feel if the situation improved. It is also useful to help patients imagine how they would feel if things did not improve. This question helps patients focus on tangible elements in the situation that must change for them to feel better.

Are you willing to take action to improve the situation for yourself? (How important is it to you for this situation to improve?) This question helps patients develop clarity about whether or not they are fully committed to changing the situation. It is a crucial question. However, for the question to have an impact, patients should feel free to make or not make a commitment to change. It is important that patients do not feel pressured to change to please the health care professional because changes made in response to such pressure seldom last.

What are some steps that you could take to bring you closer to where you want to be? (What could you do to help solve this problem? Are there any barriers you would have to overcome? Are there other people who could help you?) This question helps patients develop a specific plan that will make their commitment to change concrete. It is useful to consider the various actions that could be taken, barriers to those actions, and potential resources, personal and otherwise, that patients could use to help themselves.

Is there one thing that you will do when you leave here to improve things for yourself? This question helps patients focus on the first thing they will do to begin to improve the situation. It is useful to end the session by having identified at least one immediate step the patient will take to begin the behavior change process. It is helpful, in many situations, to write down the action so that subsequent visits can include a discussion of how the problem-solving process proceeded and new strategies that can be tried if the process was not successful. Participants in a group class can tell others in the group what they will do. Patients may wish to take a written copy of their commitment home with them. Commitments tend to be more binding when they are expressed publicly and/or documented.

If the answer to the last question is "yes," I (the patient) will:

_____

_____

_____

_____

_____

How did the plan we discussed at your last visit work out? (What happened when you tried the behavior? Why do you think that it worked (or didn't work)? What did you learn? Would you do anything differently next time? Based on this experience, what goal would you like to set for next time?)

The purpose of this question is to help patients view the behavior and the behavior change efforts as experiments. The purpose of experiments is to try something new and to learn from the experience. Whether the effort is successful or not, learning can still occur. In fact, some of our best lessons come from experiments that did not accomplish what we had planned.

In traditional care, health care professionals evaluate patient behaviors and offer positive or negative feedback based on their judgment of the patients' success or failure. When using the empowerment approach, it is essential that the patient rather than the professional evaluate the outcome. This reinforces the concept that patients are responsible for their own efforts and outcome. It also offers health care professionals the opportunity to acknowledge patient efforts rather than outcomes, which is more in line with a collaborative relationship.

CASE STUDIES

The following two case studies illustrate the traditional medical approach and the empowerment approach to helping patients change behavior. The case studies are condensed descriptions of patient-professional interactions. The actual conversations would be longer. These condensed versions are meant to illustrate how the two approaches differ. The empowerment approach may require a bit more time initially but is more likely to result in the identification of problems that are meaningful to the patient and strategies that are effective for long-term behavior change.

Case Study 1: Traditional medical model approach to behavior change

Patient: I hate this diet.

Professional: How many calories are you on?

Patient: 1,400. And I try so hard, but I just can't do it. My doctor is upset with me because I don't lose weight. I do pretty well at work all day, but then Joe comes home and wants a big dinner. And then we sit together and watch TV, and he wants me to bring him ice cream. And so I eat right along with him.

Professional: Why don't you try having your husband take a walk with you after dinner? And try frozen yogurt instead of ice cream?

Patient: I tried yogurt before and I didn't like it very much. Also, I don't think Joe will be very interested in walking every night.

Professional: Try Fruity Delight Low-Fat Yogurt. It's great. And don't be so quick to give up on Joe walking. Will you at least give it a try?

Patient: Okay.

Professional: Great! I know you can do this if you really put your mind to it.

Case Study 2: Empowerment approach to behavior change

Patient: I hate this diet.

Professional: You sound pretty upset. Why don't you tell me about it.

Patient: I try so hard to cook and eat right to lose weight and keep my blood sugar in the target range. But, my husband refuses to eat that way and makes fun of me for being fat. Then, my doctor gets upset with me for not losing weight. I made a meal plan with the dietitian and thought it would work, but I just can't use it like I want to.

Professional: That must be frustrating—to try so hard and not feel like you are getting anywhere.

Patient: It sure is. Why is it so hard for me?

Professional: What do you think the problem is?

Patient: Well, I do pretty well at work all day, but then Joe comes home and wants a big dinner. And then we sit together and watch TV, and he wants me to bring him ice cream. And so I eat right along with him.

Professional: What would have to change about this situation for you to feel better?

Patient:	You know, I really do want to lose weight. Not just because my doctor told me, but because I don't like how I look, and I don't have much energy to do the things I enjoy anymore.
Professional:	What will happen if you don't change anything?
Patient:	I'm not sure. I guess I'll gain more weight and my health will probably get worse, too.
Professional:	How will you feel if that happens?
Patient:	Awful. I'm just about at the end of my rope. I hate being frustrated and mad at myself all of the time. It's even affecting my work. And I'm crabby with the kids, too.
Professional:	Are you willing to have things stay the way they are now?
Patient:	No! I've just got to lose some weight.
Professional:	What is one thing you can do when you leave here to get you started?
Patient:	I am going to talk to Joe. I can't believe he knows how bad I feel about the things he says. If I can just get him on my side, the battle would be half over.
Professional:	When are you going to talk to him?
Patient:	Tonight, when he gets home from work.

CONCLUSION

Effective diabetes care requires new roles for both health care professionals and patients. By creating a collaborative relationship, both the health care provider and the patient can find themselves in a satisfying partnership that results in improved glycemic control for the patient and an enhanced sense of self-efficacy and level of satisfaction with care for both parties.

BIBLIOGRAPHY

Anderson RM, Funnell MM: Compliance and adherence are dysfunctional concepts in diabetes care. *Diabetes Educ* 26:597–604, 2000
Anderson RM, Funnell MM: *The Art of Empowerment: Stories and Strategies for Diabetes Educators.* Alexandria, VA, American Diabetes Association, 2000

Anderson RM, Funnell MM, Butler PM, Arnold MS, Fitzgerald JT, Feste CC: Patient empowerment: results of a randomized controlled trial. *Diabetes Care* 18:943–949, 1995

Funnell MM: Helping patients take charge of their chronic illnesses. *Fam Pract Manag* 7:47–51, 2000

Funnell MM, Anderson RM: The problem with compliance in diabetes. *JAMA* 284:1709, 2000

Funnell MM, Anderson RM: Putting Humpty Dumpty back together again: reintegrating the clinical and behavioral components in diabetes care and education. *Diabetes Spectrum* 12:19–23, 1999

Glasgow RE, Anderson RM: In diabetes care, moving from compliance to adherence is not enough: something entirely different is needed. *Diabetes Care* 22:2090–2091, 1999

Robert M. Anderson, EdD, is a Professor of Medical Education at the University of Michigan Medical School in Ann Arbor, MI. Martha M. Funnell, MS, RN, CDE, is the Director for Administration at the Michigan Diabetes Research and Training Center in Ann Arbor, MI.

2

Working with Interpersonal Styles in the Patient-Provider Relationship

PAUL CIECHANOWSKI, MD, MPH

The Diabetes Control and Complications Trial and the U.K. Prospective Diabetes Study have emphasized the importance of achieving near-normal blood glucose levels in patients with type 1 and type 2 diabetes to minimize serious long-term complications. Adhering to a strict self-care regimen (including medications, diet, and exercise) may be a challenge for the majority of diabetic patients because diabetes is one of the most psychologically and behaviorally demanding of chronic medical illnesses. As a result of this complexity, most patients with diabetes need to regularly depend on other individuals, including health care providers, for support in their diabetes self-care regimen.

UNDERSTAND THE ROLE OF THE PATIENT-PROVIDER RELATIONSHIP

Enhanced collaboration between the patient and provider has been associated with improved outcomes in chronic medical illnesses and with better treatment adherence and metabolic control in diabetes. Motivational approaches to diabetes treatment, such as self-determination theory, suggest that patients are more likely to adhere to treatment if they *perceive* that their providers understand their perspective and feelings and that their providers offer choices in treatment. A key component of such a patient-centered approach may be the provider's flexibility in attuning to a patient's unique interpersonal style—based on interpersonal needs, perceptions, and behaviors—rather than relying solely on generic "bedside manner."

Further support for improving your understanding of patients' interpersonal styles can be found in literature on challenging or difficult patients. Patient behaviors that tend to frustrate providers typically fall along a spectrum, with overuse of health care on one end of the spectrum and poor adherence to treatment and infrequent health care visits on the other. Such behaviors, which are often expressions of interpersonal needs and fears, make providers feel less effective and frustrated with the care they provide, often leading to an impasse in the treatment relationship. In fact, providers may vary considerably about which patients they perceive as "difficult." Providers who are more successful at tolerating and working with challenging patient behaviors often have developed flexible repertoires of responses that vary with patients' unique interpersonal needs and perceptions.

To improve the quality of the patient-provider relationship and, in turn, improve patient participation, negotiation, adherence to treatment, and treatment outcomes, providers need a way to rapidly and systematically assess a patient's interpersonal expectations and perceptions. This can help the provider to better understand the patient and to target effective responses to these patient characteristics. Such a step could occur before or in concert with implementation of other more traditional behavioral skills used by the provider. Assessing a patient's interpersonal style may also help to match specific behavioral or communication skills to optimize patient-provider communication. In this chapter, we present a practical way of clinically assessing and responding to patients' interpersonal styles using the construct of attachment theory.

LEARN ABOUT THE ATTACHMENT STYLE OF YOUR PATIENTS

Attachment theory can be used as a way of systematically understanding patients' perceptions of and ability to collaborate in the health care relationship—a relationship that may have more to do with patients' preexisting generalized views about relying on people than about specific behaviors of the provider at the time of a clinic visit. When developing attachment theory, John Bowlby proposed that all individuals psychologically incorporate prior experiences with caregivers, forming enduring, stable cognitive models or "maps" of caregiving that persist into adulthood. These cognitive models are learned ways of interacting in interpersonal relationships throughout life and particularly at times of vulnerability (e.g., illness). These cognitive models influence whether individuals deem themselves worthy of care and whether others are perceived as trustworthy to provide care.

Based on Bowlby's work and decades of empirical research on infants, children, and adults, Bartholomew developed a classification system for adults, outlined in Figure 2.1, that is comprised of four attachment styles: *secure, dismissing, preoccupied,* and *fearful.* Although it is possible to determine the degree to which an individual is characterized by each of these attachment styles by using continuous measures of attachment, it is often more clinically useful to determine an individual's predominant attachment style using a self-report instrument (Figure 2.2):

- Individuals with *secure* attachment likely experienced *consistently responsive* early caregiving (resulting in a positive view of self and others), and they are comfortable depending on others and are readily comforted by others.
- Individuals with *dismissing* attachment are likely to have experienced early caregiving that was *consistently unresponsive*, and in response, they adapt by becoming compulsively self-reliant. Although they are uncomfortable being close to or trusting others (negative view of others), they possess a positive view of themselves, based in large part on their self-reliance. It may be useful clinically, particularly if discussing attachment styles with patients, to use the term "self-reliant interpersonal style."
- Individuals with *preoccupied* attachment likely experienced caregiving that was *inconsistently responsive*. In an effort to ensure proximity to caregivers, they learn to habitually do more than their share in attachment relationships, becoming excessively vigilant of attachment relationships and emotionally dependent on others' approval (positive view of others), often to the point of being clingy. However, they generally have poor self-esteem, more

Model (View) of Self

		+	−
Model (View) of Other	**+**	**Secure Attachment** • Trusting of others • Feels worthy of others' attention *Clinical characteristics:* ↑ Treatment adherence ↑↓ Primary care use ↓ Symptom reporting	**Preoccupied Attachment** ("support-seeking" style) (Questionnaire style C) • Emotionally dependent on others • Low self-esteem *Clinical characteristics:* ↑↓ Treatment adherence ↑ Primary care use ↑ Symptom reporting
	−	**Dismissing Attachment** ("self-reliant" style) (Questionnaire style D) • Compulsively self-reliant • Low trust of others *Clinical characteristics:* ↓ Treatment adherence ↓ Primary care use ↑↓ Symptom reporting	**Fearful Attachment** ("cautious" style) (Questionnaire style B) • Approach-avoidance behavior • Fearful of intimacy *Clinical characteristics:* ↓ Treatment adherence ↓ Primary care use ↑ Symptom reporting

FIGURE 2.1 Attachment style categories in medical patients and model of self and others. Adapted from Bartholomew K, Horowitz LM: Attachment styles among young adults: a test of a four-category model. *J Pers Soc Psychol* 61:226–244, 1991.

subjective distress, and a significant focus on negative affect (negative view of self). It may be helpful when discussing this attachment style clinically to use a term such as "support-seeking interpersonal style."

■ Individuals with *fearful* attachment share many of the characteristics of those with *preoccupied* attachment in that they desire social contact, but this desire is ultimately inhibited by fear of rejection. These individuals are proposed to have had overly rejecting or harsh caregiving (resulting in a negative view of self and others), and, as adults, they are more likely to demonstrate interpersonal patterns in which they flee upon achieving any closeness, i.e., they exhibit approach-avoidance behavior stemming from a fear of intimacy. Like individuals with *preoccupied* attachment, they have

---

PLEASE READ THE DIRECTIONS!

Following are descriptions of four general relationship styles that people often report.

Please read each description and CIRCLE the letter corresponding to the style that *best* describes you or is *closest* to the way you generally are in your close relationships.

A. It is easy for me to become emotionally close to others. I am comfortable depending on them and having them depend on me. I don't worry about being alone or having others not accept me.

B. I am uncomfortable getting close to others. I want emotionally close relationships, but I find it difficult to trust others completely, or to depend on them. I worry that I will be hurt if I allow myself to become too close to others.

C. I want to be completely emotionally intimate with others, but I often find that others are reluctant to get as close as I would like. I am uncomfortable being without close relationships, but I sometimes worry that others don't value me as much as I value them.

D. I am comfortable without close emotional relationships. It is very important to me to feel independent and self-sufficient, and I prefer not to depend on others or have others depend on me.

FIGURE 2.2 Relationship questionnaire. Reprinted with permission from Bartholomew K, Horowitz LM: Attachment styles among young adults: a test of a four-category model. *J Pers Soc Psychol* 61:226–244, 1991.

poor self-esteem and an increased focus on negative affect. Another more readily accepted term to use clinically for this type of attachment style might be "cautious interpersonal style."

Bartholomew suggested that these individual differences in attachment patterns may have implications for communication in interpersonal relationships. For example, individuals with generalized negative perceptions of others or with a negative *other* model of attachment (dismissing and fearful attachment) have learned that people are likely to ignore or reject their attempts to gain support; therefore, they are less likely to seek support and are generally thought to have less self-disclosure and openness in relationships. Individuals with a negative *self* model of attachment (preoccupied and fearful attachment), on the other hand, are anxious about relationships and may generally be more likely to report somatic symptoms as a consequence of their tendency to focus on negative affect. This result corresponds with research suggesting that a focus on negative affect correlates with subjective health complaints, even in the absence of objective evidence of disease.

CLINICAL EXAMPLES OF INSECURE
ATTACHMENT IN PATIENTS WITH DIABETES

VIGNETTE 1: Dismissing attachment (self-reliant interpersonal style): "I prefer to not depend on others or have others depend on me."

You have not seen Ron, a 42-year-old divorced businessman with type 2 diabetes, in your primary care clinic for 4 months. As his provider, you try to schedule regular visits with Ron, but he has not kept his last two follow-up appointments. Ron comes into your office today but makes no mention of missing appointments. He requests a refill for glyburide, which he wants to restart after running out 2 months ago, and says that when he called your office for a refill, your receptionist suggested he come in because he had not been seen for an extended period. His glycated hemoglobin A1C (A1C) level was 10.7% 6 months ago. He reassures you that he is going to follow suggestions from an American Diabetes Association pamphlet for improving diet and exercise that he found today in your waiting room. He says he was taking his oral hypoglycemics "most of the time" before he ran out but was rarely checking his blood glucose because he felt it didn't make a difference. He politely interrupts you when you start talking about the importance of his coming in more frequently, announcing that he has to get back to his office and that he would appreciate a refill of medication for 6 months. You immediately feel angry and somewhat hopeless and abruptly tell him that he is not taking his diabetes seriously. You tell him you can only give him a 1-month supply of medication and that you would like to see him again before he gets a refill.

Comment: At some level of awareness, patients with dismissing attachment, like Ron, may view others as unavailable or incapable of providing care; however, as a defensive strategy, they are predominantly aware of their self-reliance and lack of need of others. Difficulties in relationships are minimized or dismissed. In the presence of noncollaborative patients with dismissing attachment, providers may feel angry, unacknowledged, incompetent, and hopeless and may unconsciously neglect to keep these patients in active treatment because of the negative feelings they arouse. Alternatively, providers may try to exert control over these patients or the situation by demanding more visits or by overemphasizing a poor prognostic course to frighten the patient into compliance. Unfortunately, these types of provider behaviors may inadvertently lead to even greater distancing by the patient.

VIGNETTE 2: Preoccupied attachment (support-seeking interpersonal style): "I often find that others are reluctant to get as close as I would like."

Jordan is a 32-year-old patient with type 1 diabetes who last saw you in your tertiary care clinic 2 weeks ago. You are surprised to see him on your schedule today because you had last scheduled him for an 8-week follow-up appointment. You ask if anything has changed since the last visit, and he tells you that he is still worried about his fatigue and concentration problems. These problems are chronic and unrelated to his glucose control, and you have reassured him previously, to the extent of working him up for various medical conditions. His A1C level last month was 8.1%, and, generally, Jordan demonstrates reasonable adherence to glucose monitoring and medication but has difficulty limiting junk food when he is emotionally distressed. He asks if you can check his A1C level again and if he can get a computed tomography scan of his head. After trying to reassure him regarding his medical complaints, you are ready to set up another appointment, at which point he tells you that he feels that your nutritionist doesn't like him because she doesn't want to see him for another 3 months. Again, you try to reassure him, realize you are late for your next patient, and begin to feel overwhelmed. You ask him to return in 4 weeks, but he tells you that he has already arranged to see you in 2 weeks.

Comment: Individuals with preoccupied attachment likely heighten their expression of attachment needs and feelings to ensure their caregiver's care and availability. They may be likely to call their providers between appointments, report numerous symptoms, and demand extra appointments. Their primary mode of relating is to be highly dependent on others. Yet from an interpersonal perspective, as we see with Jordan, these individuals paradoxically see providers as constantly being insufficiently available. Patients with preoccupied attachment evoke in providers feelings of being overwhelmed, swamped, frustrated, and angry.

VIGNETTE 3:

Fearful attachment (cautious interpersonal style): "I worry that I will be hurt if I allow myself to become too close to others."

Cory, a 42-year-old obese patient with type 2 diabetes, has not been in your clinic for 6 months. You are surprised to see her in the waiting room because, over that period of time, she has made four appointments but has kept none until today. A review of her automated records over 3 years shows small clusters of visits every several months, at which time she reluctantly reports various bodily symptoms and at which time there appears to be a crisis in her life. She lives alone and works as a freelance stage set designer for numerous theater companies, since she prefers to limit her work on a job site to only several weeks before moving to a new set. Unfortunately, without a consistent employer, she is unable to get good medical insurance. Her last A1C level was 10.2%. She requests refills for her oral hypoglycemic agents. You realize that she had received only a 3-month supply of medication at her last visit and assume that she has been getting care elsewhere. She acknowledges getting her oral hypoglycemics refilled once at an urgent care clinic but states that the medical bill she received after that visit made her think twice about getting medication there again. She reassures you that she will take her medication this time, but you feel doubtful and frustrated.

Comment: Individuals with fearful attachment may have a tendency to make appointments, particularly when distressed, that they ultimately do not show up for. They have a profound inability to trust others and are extremely sensitive to any signs of rejection. Despite generally experiencing high levels of distress and physical symptoms, patients with fearful attachment, like Cory, are generally inhibited in how much they disclose to providers, making providers feel frustrated and hopeless. Again, as with patients who have dismissing attachment, providers may try to exert control over patients with fearful attachment with demands for more visits or by overemphasizing a dire prognostic course to frighten the patient into compliance. Such measures are likely to confirm the expectations of these patients that the patient-provider relationship is perilous.

LEARN ABOUT YOUR ATTACHMENT STYLE AS A PROVIDER

Providers, like patients, have varying degrees of adverse caregiving experiences and losses, and the extent to which they have come to terms with these situations vary. It is likely that the prevalence of insecure attachment among health care providers is approximately that of the national norm; a large epidemiological survey, the National Comorbidity Survey, found that approximately 41% of the general population has insecure attachment. Insecure attachment in providers or patients may contribute to less effective health care communication. In a study assessing attachment style in providers, Dozier et al. found that securely attached providers were able to hear and respond to underlying dependency needs of patients with dismissing attachment to a greater degree than insecurely attached providers, who were more likely to make superficial interventions and to be less available to these patients. When working with patients with preoccupied attachment, insecurely attached providers were more likely to perceive and attend to patients' overt dependency rather than underlying needs. Clinicians can get a better sense of their own attachment style by completing an attachment style questionnaire (Figure 2.2). Clinicians need not be put off if they match predominantly in one of the "insecure" attachment categories. In fact, having a self-reliant style, for example, may provide advantages in fulfilling the demanding work schedule of a health care provider. However, the clinician can use this information for reflecting on which areas to develop interpersonally so as to increase his or her flexibility of responses with various patient interpersonal styles.

USE ATTACHMENT THEORY AS A STRATEGY TO IMPROVE PATIENT-PROVIDER RELATIONSHIPS

We can use attachment theory to improve the patient-provider relationship in the diabetes setting in three ways: *1*) by increasing provider awareness of patient and provider attachment styles, *2*) by using clinic triage and population-based approaches, and *3*) by using problem-solving approaches and role-playing. Based on generally established population-based and behavioral principles and interventions, these approaches also make clinical use of a short self-report instrument (Figure 2.2), which can establish the attachment style of those patients who have indications of significant nonadherence or who demonstrate extreme health care use. Whereas high health care use in patients with preoccupied attachment may be overwhelming to the clinician, these interventions will generally focus on patients with dismissing and fearful attachment, since research has shown these patients may be more likely to minimize coordinated health care visits (possibly leading to delays in timely health care seeking or use of uncoordinated health care, such as emergency room or urgent care visits) or demonstrate poor adherence with diabetes self-care regimens.

Benefits of Increasing Provider Awareness of Attachment Styles

- Less disparaging developmental formulations of patients' perspectives and behaviors may begin to replace an overemphasis on labeling patient behaviors as difficult or challenging.
- Identifying the patient's interpersonal style may lead to increased empathy and tolerance of challenging patient behaviors, thus minimizing the likelihood of an impasse resulting from provider frustration.
- Awareness of attachment styles may lead to increased self-awareness and reflection on the providers' own role in unsatisfying patient-provider relationships.

Uses of Clinic Triage and Population-Based Approaches Based on Attachment Styles

For patients with dismissing and fearful attachment:

- Providing good care on the patient's terms may mean accepting patient's attachment style (e.g., fear of intimacy or low trust of others). Practically, this may mean decreasing the relative threat of intimacy within a clinical setting by having a small number of providers in the clinic alternating to provide coordinated care.
- Population-based tracking using automated data, telephone calls, and appointments conducted over the telephone, as well as proactive reminders/contacts may all be required to prevent these patients from falling through the cracks.
- Using principles of empowerment (see Chapter 1) or motivational interviewing techniques may help the provider to work collabora-

tively with the patient with dismissing attachment without threatening the patient's compulsive need for self-reliance.

For patients with preoccupied attachment:

- Frequent, regularly scheduled, brief visits with a consistent provider will help to extinguish high health care use and excessive use of emergency room and urgent care visits. As an example, 20- to 30-min weekly sessions that focus on both medical and psychosocial aspects of care can be carried out, with strict limits on length of visit and reasonably strict limits on between-session communication.

Relationship-Focused Problem-Solving and Role-Play

Problem-solving

Patients vary in the degree to which their behavior is dictated by less flexible insecure attachment styles. Therefore, short-term problem-solving approaches that focus on attachment style may be attempted with most patients.

- Disengaged patients with dismissing or fearful attachment can be asked to generate a list of diabetes self-care behaviors under columns labeled "high relationship-dependent" (e.g., diet) or "low relationship-dependent" (e.g., glucose monitoring) to determine which self-care behaviors the patient perceives could benefit from improved collaboration with others (e.g., family, spouse, friends, providers). Patients may also generate a separate list of ideas about why they don't trust important others or providers in general.
- With the help of the provider, patients can brainstorm and generate lists of solutions for overcoming barriers and improving interactions with others when carrying out "high relationship-dependent" self-care activities.
- Any potential solutions that the patient conceives of should be considered, but one simple, practical solution that has the highest probability of succeeding should be picked as homework to be carried out before the next session. For example, a patient may determine that to succeed in following a daily walking regimen, he or she could either call an acquaintance who is also interested in walking to lose weight or enroll in a fitness club that focuses on

walking. After considering the pros and cons of each approach, the patient may decide that the walking club would be preferable because it would not require as much camaraderie, and the goal for the week would be to make phone contact to enroll with the fitness club.

Role-play

- The provider and patient may role-play to explore interpersonal barriers and try out solutions that the patient has come up with. Such role-playing will help patients trigger thoughts or feelings about important barriers preventing them from making contact with providers or family members.
- By switching roles, patients will be able to try out and experience the perspectives of significant others, family members, or providers. For example, the provider can play the part of the patient, and ask the patient to play the part of the diabetes clinician or a concerned spouse. By discussing a specific self-care issue, such as medication taking or meal preparation, patients can discover a tremendous amount about how their self-care issues are perceived by others or how their own perceptions of barriers to optimal self-care may not be totally accurate, particularly as pertains to the social dimension of such self-care behaviors.

Assessing Family Support

When appropriate, assessment and feedback about current family and support network patterns pertaining to diabetes self-care (e.g., meal planning) may be explored as well. This is best approached with the patient by normalizing and showing the adaptivity of the specific attachment style in the past and in other domains of life while emphasizing the importance of reliance on others in achieving good outcomes in chronic illnesses such as diabetes. For example, a patient with dismissing attachment may be told the following: "Individuals with high self-reliance are often able to accomplish a lot in their lives. In fact, self-reliance is highly valued in our society. However, research has repeatedly shown that working with others—such as family members, significant others, and health care providers—is extremely important in individuals with chronic illnesses such as diabetes." Where appropriate, providing such nonthreatening feedback with significant others present may lead to improved outcomes, since family members may inevitably be part of the interpersonal web that may otherwise reinforce a patient's inflexible interpersonal approach to managing his or her diabetes self-care. An assessment of attachment patterns in the family is best done while considering other aspects of the family system covered in Chapter 19.

CONCLUSION

There are many factors that determine whether the patient-provider relationship is a collaborative one, including demographic and cultural match, medical comorbidity, and factors related to the health care setting. Nevertheless, to effectively collaborate with patients, particularly those with suboptimal diabetes self-management, the provider will certainly benefit from a better understanding of interpersonal styles and should recognize several principles:

- Good bedside manner is typically not sufficient in effectively communicating with patients who are disengaged from or over-reliant upon the health care relationship.
- On an emotional level, the patient-provider relationship may recapitulate earlier caregiving relationships.
- Relatively inflexible and reflexive ideas about being cared for (e.g., issues of trust and self-worth) may determine, in large part, observable health behaviors such as frequency of health care visits and adherence to diabetes self-care.
- Providers can optimize patient-provider communication by better understanding their own interpersonal style and their patients' interpersonal styles, leading to a broader clinical repertoire of responses to a patient's unique interpersonal style and needs.

Attachment theory provides an important framework for understanding the behaviors and perceptions of patients and providers when they come together in a clinical setting. Incorporating attachment theoretical principles into medical care of patients with diabetes will lead to a better understanding of patients and sound approaches for intervening with patients who may present with suboptimal diabetes self-management.

ACKNOWLEDGMENTS

This work and preparation of this chapter were supported by National Institutes of Health Grant DK60652-01, by Group Health Cooperative/Kaiser Permanente Community Foundation Grant 66-0404, and by Bayer Institute for Health Care Communication Grant 98-439.

BIBLIOGRAPHY

Bartholomew K: From childhood to adult relationships: attachment theory and research. In *Understanding Relationship Processes 2: Learning About Relationships.* Duck S, Ed. Beverly Hills, CA, Sage Publications, 1993, pp. 30–62

Bartholomew K, Horowitz LM: Attachment styles among young adults: a test of a four-category model. *J Pers Soc Psychol* 61:226–244, 1991

Bowlby J: *Attachment and Loss. Volume II: Separation: Anxiety and Anger.* New York, Basic Books, 1973

Ciechanowski PS, Hirsch IB, Katon WJ: Interpersonal predictors of HbA$_{1c}$ in patients with type 1 diabetes. *Diabetes Care* 25:731–736, 2002

Ciechanowski PS, Katon WJ, Russo JE, Walker EA: The patient-provider relationship: attachment theory and adherence to treatment in diabetes. *Am J Psychiatry* 158:29–35, 2001

Ciechanowski PS, Walker EA, Katon WJ, Russo JE: Attachment theory: a model for health care utilization and somatization. *Psychosomatic Medicine.* In press

Dozier M, Cue KL, Barnett L: Clinicians as caregivers: role of attachment organization in treatment. *J Cons Clin Psych* 62:793–800, 1994

Mickelson KD, Kessler RC, Shaver PR: Adult attachment in a nationally representative sample. *J Pers Soc Psychol* 73:1092–1106, 1997

Williams GC, Freedman ZR, Deci EL: Supporting autonomy to motivate patients with diabetes for glucose control. *Diabetes Care* 21:1644–1651, 1998

Paul Ciechanowski, MD, MPH, is an Assistant Professor of Consultation-Liaison & Primary Care Psychiatry in the Department of Psychiatry & Behavioral Sciences at the University of Washington in Seattle, WA.

3

Understanding and Treating Professional Burnout

CINDY L. HANSON, PhD

A growing number of people are experiencing emotional and physical exhaustion as a result of work overload. The demands for increased productivity with less resources and reduced budgets have strained many organizations, and the effects of this stress have become apparent in professional burnout. The misconception that the burnout process merely reflects individual weaknesses (e.g., a weak character or poor attitude) often clouds the major organizational changes that are necessary to prevent burnout. There are some strategies, however, geared to the individual level, that are useful in preventing professional burnout.

Although the process of burnout starts at the organizational level and is felt at the individual level, knowing the organizational stressors and changes that can precipitate burnout is helpful in identifying and initiating the changes to alleviate it. Many of the organizational stressors that lead to burnout include work overload, conflicting individual and organizational values, insufficient rewards, a reduced sense of organizational cohesiveness, distrust in the fairness of an organization, and the increased demand for services without adequate resources for support. Several of these stressors are accentuated in health care environments because of the emotionally demanding nature of the work. Effective diabetes management requires considerable energy and endurance from providers as well as patients. Successful diabetes management involves individualized self-care goals, persistent problem-solving efforts, and ongoing provider support. Despite concerted efforts, treatment outcomes may fall short of expectations. Patients and providers can reciprocally reinforce feelings of disappointment, frustration, and failure, and this process can perpetuate burnout in both the patient and provider. Provider burnout disrupts an important therapeutic alliance.

Several guidelines are discussed in this chapter:

- Learn about professional burnout
- Know the signs of professional burnout
- Understand the causes of professional burnout
- Practice strategies to prevent or reverse professional burnout

LEARN ABOUT PROFESSIONAL BURNOUT

Burnout can be conceptualized as a gradual downward spiral from work strains at the organizational level, leading to emotional and physical manifestations in the provider (e.g., drop in quality and quantity of work, increased work-related conflicts, and physical exhaustion). Burnout consists of psychological and physical responses to chronic job stressors that occur frequently in the caregiving, helping, or people-oriented professions. The chronic job stressors often involve *1*) unrealistic job expectations and demands and *2*) unreciprocated caregiving in emotionally draining and stressful situations. Burnout is reflected in the following negative changes in provider attitudes and behaviors as a result of chronic interpersonal and emotional stress at work:

- A state of physical, emotional, and mental exhaustion
- A progressive loss of idealism, energy, and purpose
- Feelings of helplessness and hopelessness, emotional drain, negative self-concept, and negative attitudes toward work, life, and people
- Depletion of physical and mental resources by excessively striving to reach unrealistic expectations imposed by yourself or by the values of others

Professional burnout generally results in a drain of provider energy and an inability to respond effectively to the demands of the job.

KNOW THE SIGNS OF PROFESSIONAL BURNOUT

Signs of professional burnout usually involve one or more of the following:

- Emotional exhaustion
- Depersonalization
- Reduced personal accomplishments

Emotional exhaustion refers to feelings of being emotionally overextended and depleted. Providers who work more hours and have overly excessive time demands are more likely to experience emotional exhaustion and feelings such as frustration and irritation. Providers who are emotionally exhausted may try to reduce or minimize contact with patients. This provider-patient distancing can create feelings in patients of provider negligence and nonsupport (see Chapter 2). Providers who are emotionally and physically drained are less able to help their patients.

Depersonalization refers to the impersonal and insensitive responses of providers who develop burnout. Provider attitudes can become callous, and providers may act rude to staff and patients. This "closes down" people rather than "building them up," and it hurts the provider-patient relationship, which further contributes to patient and provider burnout. Providers may depersonalize patients because of failures in treatment or because of discomfort with the feelings and needs of patients. Providers may become less sensitive when patients are experiencing failures and difficulties, which is when the patients' needs are highest. Moreover, providers who feel professionally defeated are more likely to blame patients for poor health outcomes—another way of depersonalizing and distancing patients. Providers who have "tuned out" patients may not understand the patients' difficulties or detect the need for appropriate referrals.

Reduced personal accomplishment occurs when the provider withdraws and is unable to meet the demands of the job. The provider may withdraw from job demands to maintain a sense of control and preserve whatever resources and energy remain. A sense of incompetence and feelings of failure further escalate the burnout process. Some providers do not experience a reduced sense of personal accomplishment in work as part of the burnout process, although they may experience a lowered sense of personal accomplishment and success in family and other social networks.

UNDERSTAND THE CAUSES OF PROFESSIONAL BURNOUT

Few research studies exist on burnout among providers who care for people with diabetes. In the wider literature, a few consistent patterns emerge as predictors of professional burnout. Burnout results from a combination of interrelated factors:

- High job-related stresses (e.g., overcommitment, lack of staff support, inadequate funding and institutional support, low control over work demands, lack of job security)
- Low satisfaction in work and interpersonal relationships (e.g., dissatisfaction with work load, emotional exhaustion, poor relationships with colleagues and staff, low support from family and friends)
- Caregiving to patients with chronic or severe debilitating problems

In addition to the organizational stressors mentioned above, burnout is more likely to develop in providers who care for patients with diabetes when the following occur:

- Unrealistic patient and provider goals and expectations have been set
- A consistent and positive approach has not been used (nor modeled to patients) by providers
- Too much responsibility for the ongoing support and problem-solving has been undertaken by the provider, and appropriate referrals and resources have not been identified or have been underused

PRACTICE STRATEGIES TO PREVENT OR REVERSE BURNOUT

Just as the road to burnout reflects a *continuum* of negative changes, many of which may be outside the control of the individual involved, the road to renewed invigoration, creativity, and job satisfaction entails a healing *process* that occurs over time. Importantly, the provider needs to:

- Set realistic short- and long-term goals for self and patient
- Be sensitive to his or her own feelings, beliefs, attitudes, and biases
- Be open to appropriate feedback from caring family and friends
- Identify developmental life changes and demands for self and patient
- Balance priorities for self and with patients
- Operate under the premise that the primary task of the provider is not to be the sole provider, but rather to help the patient develop a professional and personal support network
- Engage familial or other support systems
- Develop a team approach to care with referral sources
- Use community resources for diabetes-related and lifestyle support

These prevention strategies are outlined in more detail below:

1. Set realistic short- and long-term goals for self, and set goals for patients that allow for normal fluctuations in disease management throughout the course of the patient's life. Both patients and providers need to recognize small successes and be prepared for the chronicity of the disease and the demands that are placed on patients and providers. Providers who ask patients what goals they wish to achieve and help devise specific plans to obtain only one or two of these goals are more likely to experience patient success than burnout. Understanding the additional health and life demands placed on patients, as well as the patient's ability to cope with these multiple daily health tasks and expectations, helps the provider set realistic and achievable short-term goals. Long-term goals are achieved with short-term successes.

2. Be sensitive to your own feelings, beliefs, attitudes, and biases and be open to feedback from caring family and friends. With professional burnout, the provider not only becomes less sensitive to the patient, but also becomes less aware of his or her own feelings of disengagement, which undermine treatment efforts. Colleagues often experience similar stressful work demands and may share "blind spots" regarding the emotional and physical costs of chronic work stress on the clinician and others. When providers experience burnout, treatment efforts that are most successful in changing patients' lifestyles (ongoing support and mutual patient-provider problem-solving) are impaired. Family members and friends can help the provider recognize the effects of the escalating stress. The provider can then identify those areas that are contributing to the problem and seek solutions.

3. Identify developmental life changes and demands necessary in setting appropriate expectations, recognizing sources of stress, and providing anticipatory guidance to patients. Patients' ways of coping with diabetes shift with different developmental tasks and life milestones. If the provider understands some of the developmental tasks facing patients, he or she will be better able to set realistic expectations, provide appropriate anticipatory guidance to patients, and help avoid patient and provider burnout. From a developmental perspective, it is also important for the provider to recognize that he or she may experience a reevaluation of life goals and career choice in mid-life or after 10–15 years in practice. During this readjustment period, problems associated with provider burnout, occupational stress, and job dissatisfaction may be intensified.

4. Balance priorities for self and with patients. To avoid burnout, providers who have heavy and demanding schedules need to care for their own physical and emotional health and to pace themselves so that their work is balanced with other sources of support and pleasure. Providers need to distinguish between urgent demands and important life priorities to make wise choices regarding balancing their time. Providers can help patients prioritize their life demands to maximize their health outcomes. People require rest and relaxation to be rejuvenated and perform at optimal levels. Without balance, people eventually fall ill emotionally, relationally, and/or physically. In Japan, the term *karoshi* describes professionals who die suddenly because of overwork.

5. Operate under the premise that the primary task of the provider is not to be the sole provider but rather to help the patient develop a support network. (See points 6–8 below.)

6. Engage familial or other support systems for providers and patients. Support is an important predictor of healthy years of life and is an important buffer to stress. Providers and patients, as well as family members and friends, need to identify what types of support the patient or provider desires, when the support is needed (e.g., at home, at work), and how often the provider or patient desires the supportive behaviors (see Chapter 19). Even small steps to increase the supportive environment and pleasurable activities for providers and/or patients can make a big difference.

7. Develop a team approach to care with referral sources. A consistent factor that emerges in the literature to help prevent professional burnout is having collaborative support from other professionals. Ideally, a team approach is useful in managing the multiple and complex treatment demands of diabetes and the support needed by the patient and family. If the team approach is unavailable, the provider can consult with other professionals to build a network of referral sources. Sharing provider-patient experiences and problems with other providers can also help to alleviate work stress and often provides new insights into solving ongoing problems. Colleagues can help identify difficulties in the patients' lives to which the provider may have become insensitive and suggest solutions. Mentoring interns can also be helpful because they often generate fresh ideas and help with the workload. They also provide an avenue for the professional to feel appreciated and become more engaged at work. Having colleagues for professional support is important in preventing or treating provider burnout.

8. Use community resources for diabetes-related and lifestyle support. Table 3.1 is a list of diabetes-related national websites that may be useful in finding information on local community resources for individuals with diabetes.

CONCLUSION

Providers of diabetes care are especially vulnerable to professional burnout, and provider burnout can negatively influence patient-provider interaction. To prevent and treat professional burnout, diabetes clinicians need to know the causes and signs of professional burnout, be sensitive to their own feelings and attitudes, and understand the central role of support (for both clinicians and patients) in a disease as complex

TABLE 3.1 Diabetes-Related National Websites

American Diabetes Association	www.diabetes.org; customerservice@diabetes.org	1-800-342-2383
Juvenile Diabetes Research Foundation	www.jdrf.org; info@jdrf.org	1-800-533-2873
American Association for Diabetes Educators	www.aadenet.org; aade@aadenet.org	1-800-832-6874
National Institute of Diabetes and Digestive and Kidney Diseases	www.niddk.nih.gov	1-800-860-8747
National Diabetes Education Program	www.ndep.nih.gov	1-800-438-5383
National Diabetes Information Clearinghouse	www.niddk.nih.gov/health/diabetes/diabetes.htm; ndic@info.niddk.nih.gov	1-800-860-8747
National Kidney and Urologic Diseases Information Clearinghouse	www.niddk.nih.gov/health/kidney/kidney.htm; nkudic@info.niddk.nih.gov	1-800-891-5390
Weight-Control Information Network	www.niddk.nih.gov/health/nutrit/nutrit.htm; win@info.niddk.nih.gov	1-877-946-4627

as diabetes. Reducing or preventing professional burnout will help build the type of partnership between provider and patient that is needed to effectively manage diabetes.

BIBLIOGRAPHY

Hanson CL: The health of children with IDDM: a shift to family-centered, community-based care. *Diabetes Spectrum* 7:390–392, 1994

Maslach C: Stress, burnout, and workaholism. In *Professionals in Distress: Issues, Syndromes, and Solutions in Psychology.* Kilburg RR, Nathan PE, Thoreson RW, Eds. Washington, DC, American Psychological Association, 1986, pp. 53–75

Maslach C, Leiter MP: *The Truth About Burnout: How Organizations Cause Personal Stress and What To Do About It.* San Francisco, CA, Jossey-Bass, 1997

McKegney CP: Surviving survivors: coping with caring for patients who have been victimized. *Primary Care* 20:481–494, 1993

Musick JL: How close are you to burnout? Learn how to control stress before stress controls you. *Family Practice Management*, Vol. 4, April, 1997

Reinhold BB: *Toxic Work: How To Overcome Stress, Overload, and Burnout and Revitalize Your Career.* New York, Plume, 1997

Snibbe JR, Radcliffe T, Weisberger C, Richards M, Kelly J: Burnout among primary care physicians and mental health professionals in a managed health care setting. *Psychol Reports* 65:775–780, 1989

Cindy L. Hanson, PhD, is a clinical psychologist in Mt. Pleasant, SC.

4

Tailoring Diabetes Education and Care to Minority Patients and Families

ROBIN NWANKWO, MPH, RD, CDE
AND TRICIA S. TANG, PhD

The art of diabetes education and care is in the delivery and effectiveness. Among clinicians, nurses, educators, and other health care professionals working with and caring for patients with diabetes, the greatest challenge is delivering education and patient care in a manner meaningful to each patient. Although the biomedical aspects of diabetes are similar across patients, the experience of having diabetes can be vastly different, especially among minority communities. Given that minority communities bear a greater burden of diabetes and its complications, it is critical for health care providers to better understand the specific educational needs and issues for these patients. It should be noted that economic circumstances play a key role in diabetes self-management because they relate to health care access, use, and delivery. Because minority groups are disproportionately represented in economically disadvantaged communities, providers should consider the economic circumstance of all patients. By "walking into" the cultural lives and belief systems of our minority patients, families, and communities, we can form more collaborative partnerships, optimize care, and improve their diabetes experience.

The purpose of this chapter is to present issues that may be of particular importance for minority patients and to equip diabetes professionals with effective strategies to integrate diabetes care within the

37

unique cultural context of each patient. This chapter discusses four issues to consider when treating patients from minority communities: *1)* cultural perceptions of diabetes, *2)* the role of family in diabetes, *3)* health and illness orientation, and *4)* establishing trust and enhancing communication. Whereas these four issues are present at some level for any diabetes patient, they are especially prominent in the diabetes experience among minority patients. For each topic area, we will present the particular issue, describe how it relates to the diabetes experience, and recommend strategies for diabetes professionals to incorporate these issues into diabetes care.

ASSESS THE PATIENT'S CULTURAL PERCEPTION OF DIABETES

Cultural values and beliefs help shape our perceptions of health and illness. How patients understand the causes, symptoms, and treatment of illness guides their behaviors and management of the illness. Patients from diverse cultural backgrounds may embrace a different framework of health and medicine. As health care providers, understanding patients' perception of diabetes arms us with a common language to explain symptoms, provide education, and deliver treatment recommendations.

For example, a cultural framework of health and illness held by several minority communities is the concept of balance. According to this framework, health is a state of equilibrium. Illness develops when this harmony is disrupted, resulting in a state of excess or deficiency. In the case of diabetes, patients who embrace this health orientation may view diabetes as a condition of excess sugar or stress. Among people from some Hispanic cultures, there is a belief that eating salty foods may compensate for sugar in the body. By framing diabetes as an imbalance of "sugar" and insulin and then presenting self-management behaviors (e.g., diet, exercise, medications) as a way of restoring balance, health care providers can offer an explanation culturally consistent for these patients.

Kleinman's explanatory model is an effective tool providers can use to assess patients' personal understanding of diabetes (Table 4.1). This model consists of a series of eight questions that can be applied to minority patients regardless of cultural, ethnic, economic, social, spiritual, and geographic background. Responses to these questions will

TABLE 4.1 Kleinman's Explanatory Model

Provider questions	What patient responses tell the health care provider
What do you think caused your problem?	• Is the cause biologically, spiritually, emotionally-based? • External or internal source? • Related to God's will, patient's behavior, environment, etc.?
Why do you think it started when it did?	• Does patient believe diabetes is associated with a critical event?
What do you think your sickness does to you? How does it work?	• Patient's interpretation of what diabetes does to him or her • What symptoms patient identifies related to the diabetes • Meaning patient attaches to symptoms
How severe is your sickness? Will it have a long or short course?	• Does patient believe it is a chronic, lifelong illness or something that can be cured with the appropriate treatment? • Patient's perception of seriousness—may explain current self-management behaviors or lack thereof
What kind of treatment do you think you should receive?	• Types of treatments patient believes will be effective • Is patient willing to use pharmacological approaches? • Does patient embrace alternative approaches? • Is patient willing to use both Western and alternative approaches?
What are the most important results you hope to receive from this treatment?	• Specific areas of life patient prioritizes as important • Symptoms and issues that are of less concern for patient
What are the chief problems your sickness has caused for you?	• Most distressing symptoms for patient—providers can leverage treatment goals
What do you fear most about your illness?	• Quality of life as defined by the patient

inform providers of the optimal approach to framing diabetes education, treatment, and management with patients.

Assess Cultural Approaches to Diabetes Care

It is important to learn about the home remedies or traditional healing practices patients are using to treat their diabetes or symptoms. If patients are using self-prescribed treatments, determine whether these practices conflict with self-management behaviors. For example, practicing Qi Gong (a traditional Chinese form of movement and meditation) as a regular exercise activity is usually consistent with appropriate diabetes care. Having determined that a cultural practice is safe, a more collaborative relationship can be promoted by encouraging patients to continue these practices. Alternatively, patients may observe a cultural tradition that conflicts with diabetes care. For instance, among individuals of Muslim faith, Ramadan is a holiday of month-long consecration and fasting until sundown. Although exceptions can be made for people diagnosed with certain health conditions, if patients choose to observe the tradition, the risk of fasting hypoglycemia or hyperglycemia after fasting is significant. The provider can assist in adjusting insulin/medication doses to enhance safety.

Assess the Meaning of Diabetes in the Patient's Community

A diagnosis of diabetes may carry different connotations across cultural groups. For some minority cultures, a diabetes diagnosis reflects a personal failure of consuming excess calories, behaving immorally, or being unspiritual. Among men of some Latino cultures, diabetes is thought to result in impotency. Men who adopt this belief may hide their condition from their spouse and family and, in doing so, opt out of valuable sources of social support. Cooking is traditionally the job of the Latino wife. Wives have been reported to blame themselves for causing their husbands diabetes, creating a dynamic that detracts from an important supportive environment. Other beliefs that have potentially deleterious effects are those that categorize diabetes as a condition that cannot be prevented and controlled or an illness that deserves public ridicule or shame. Regardless of the specific beliefs, values attached to a diabetes diagnosis can serve as powerful deterrents or facilitators of diabetes care and management behaviors. Listed below are ways to assess the meaning of diabetes in the patient's life.

- What does having diabetes mean to you?
- What does having diabetes mean in your family?
- What does having diabetes mean in your community?

UNDERSTAND THE ROLE OF FAMILY IN THE PATIENT'S DIABETES CARE

For many cultures, family can play a significant role in health-related decisions. Depending on the prescribed roles and relationships observed in different cultures, patients and their families approach decision-making differently. Some cultures defer important decisions to elders in the family or community, whereas others view decisions as a group process involving all family members. For example, an African-American husband may insist on traditionally higher-fat dishes similar to those prepared by his mother. Wives may succumb to the pressure to avoid the ridicule of family, including the in-laws. Given the range of decision-making practices families and cultural communities observe, it is critical for providers to inquire about the role of family and decision-making styles for every patient (Table 4.2).

INVOLVE FAMILY AND COMMUNITY IN DIABETES CARE

Family and community support is crucial for some patients to succeed in challenging tasks such as following a diabetes regimen (e.g., diet, exercise). Patients may feel isolated when adopting new behaviors or diets. If health-promoting activities are initiated within the broader community, patients will have a wider support network. For example, without labeling activities as treatment for diabetes, some communities have initiated walking clubs, craft classes, and community-based healthy food stores as ways to improve their diet, exercise, and lower stress. Health-promoting activities may differ across cultural generations, with first-generation members embracing the traditions of their home country and latter generations more acculturated to Western cultures and practices. Therefore, initiating traditional activities, such as traditional dance classes (e.g., salsa) or drumming, will promote diabetes self-management behaviors for all members of minority communities.

TABLE 4.2 How to Assess Decision-Making Styles of Minority Patients and Their Families

• Ask patients whether they prefer other family members to be present during diabetes care and treatment discussions
• Ask patients and families their preferred approach to decision-making
• Avoid requiring patients and their families to make on-the-spot decisions
• Allow patients sufficient time to present issues/situations to their family
• Ask patients and/or their families what are the best times to discuss issues
• Consider offering family sessions
• Offer options and allow patients and/or their families to identify their preferences

Integrate Treatment Planning in the Context of Family

In many minority groups, family dynamics will have an impact on how patients incorporate new strategies for self-care. In some cases, without hesitation, needs of the family will supercede the patient's self-care needs. Suggesting simple step-by-step methods allows the patient to incorporate changes gradually without disrupting the family routine. Challenges and pressures from family members may discourage patients from engaging in self-care behaviors (e.g., reducing consumption of fatty foods). For some Latino families, the recommendation to change their diet may be interpreted as needing to buy special and expensive foods that would be unpalatable to their family. Providers can assist patients in preparing for these situations by role-playing how to address, confront, or persuade family members regarding specific issues (see Chapter 19). These exercises will equip patients with the useful skills to achieve success. In turn, patients will be empowered to set priorities for their own diabetes care.

Patients who are in the role of caregiver and head-of-household may need practice in soliciting support from family members. Will the patient allow family members to step up to be supportive? Hold a discussion on how support is needed for emergency situations such as a hypoglycemia event, and help your patient to develop a plan that includes empowering the family to take action. These situations may run counter to the prescribed roles in the family. However, with good preparation, family members can take lifesaving actions in a way that is respectful of family dynamics. Finally, continue to educate patients and their families on discordant beliefs about diabetes.

ASSESS ATTITUDES TOWARD PREVENTION

Patients' orientation toward preventive versus crisis health behavior can influence self-care habits such as exercise, medication regimes, blood glucose monitoring, and diet. Several studies show that even though African Americans embrace the importance of self-care, are willing to accept diabetes, are responsive to their health care providers, and accept their responsibility in self-care, they still report a powerlessness to prevent diabetes-related complications. This powerlessness can negatively affect their diabetes self-management. Other health orientations or attitudes that contradict the preventive goals of diabetes self-management include:

- Self-blaming attitudes when experiencing poor health
- "Live in the now" attitude
- A belief that a higher power is in control of health, not oneself

Patients who embrace these orientations may be less likely to engage in preventive behaviors such as retinopathy screening, foot care, and routine physical examinations. Although some of these beliefs need to be challenged gradually, providers can frame diabetes care in a way that complements some orientations. For patients with strong spiritual beliefs, providers can describe diabetes self-management tools as provisions made available by the powerful Other to assist the patient or explain that diabetes professionals are working through the hands of a higher power. In other words, craft messages to meet the belief system, not to change it. An example would be to say, "Man has been given wisdom to provide treatment. We are grateful for these options that can improve the quality of our life and help us to continue to serve and contribute to each other."

Promoting Prevention Within the Context of the Patient's Priorities

Making multiple lifestyle changes at once can overwhelm any patient. Providers can get their foot in the door by suggesting a single behavior change that reflects a patient's priority (see Chapter 1). What contributes to the patient's quality of life will determine his or her priorities (see Chapter 20). For example, if a patient's favorite pastime is playing ma-jong (a Chinese game that relies on good eyesight to discriminate characters on playing tiles), then framing retinopathy screening as insurance for playing ma-jong for years to come may be more persuasive than a stand-alone recommendation. Alternatively, discussing weight loss to reduce insulin resistance in a Hispanic patient whose culture values obesity as an indication of health and wealth, especially if compounded by a fatalistic belief about diabetes, would not be effective.

FOSTER TRUST AND OPEN COMMUNICATION

Diabetes care involves the relationship between two cultures—the culture of the patient and the culture of Western medicine (e.g., health care providers, health care system). Although issues of trust and communication can act as barriers between patients and the Western health care system in general, among minority patients, these barriers are even more pronounced.

Establishing a trusting relationship with minority patients proves more challenging given the history of medicine and racism that follows many patients into every health care interaction. Reluctance to seek health care because of existing negative attitudes toward Western medicine may be compounded further by conflicts in language and culture. For example, 54% of Asian elders are not proficient in the English language. Having professional interpreters available in hospitals and clinics will not only improve communication but also facilitate diabetes care and education overall. Providers and health care environments can also foster culturally supportive environments by displaying linguistically and culturally specific educational materials in waiting rooms and offices for their minority patients.

Health care professionals have adopted several approaches to improving communication with minority patients. One approach is learning about specific cultural beliefs, practices, and interpersonal communication styles of different cultural groups through books, workshops, and other training forums. The problem with this approach is that providers tend to apply these popular beliefs, traditions, and communication styles without having first explored the unique social and cultural context of patients and their families. In fact, participants representing African, Hispanic, and European American cultural groups report a preference toward services and programs tailored to individual families more so than focusing on culturally specific group needs. Once the intervention is tailored to the individual needs of the family, issues of the patients' cultural background and social circumstances can then be addressed.

Building trust and enhancing communication with minority patients relies more on an open attitude of learning and asking questions than on mastering cultural trivia of different minority communities.

Practice Cultural Humility

Cultural humility is an interpersonal stance in which providers walk into every clinical interaction with a willingness to learn from the patient about his or her cultural background and diabetes experience. For example, a provider may say, "I am not familiar with that cultural practice. Can you tell me more about it?"

Validate the Patient's Cultural Experience Related to Diabetes Care

Minority patients may adopt alternative approaches to treating or coping with diabetes. If these approaches do not conflict with diabetes care, then acknowledging or encouraging the use of these approaches facilitates a partnership with patients. For instance, patients who have a strong spiritual orientation and belief in a powerful Other may resonate with treatment rationales that describe diabetes self-management as adjunct to their preferred practices. If practices do conflict with diabetes care, then state the options and expected outcomes, empowering the patient to make an informed decision. An example would be a preference to seek a tribal healer for treating a diabetes-related illness or use of home remedies including teas and aloe. Both of these options provide fewer barriers to care than Westernized health care. After acknowledging these preferences, the provider could teach the patient to closely monitor the effect of the treatment with self–blood glucose monitors and inform the patient of what to watch for if there is limited improvement or of any contraindications of herbal remedies with current medication.

Inquire About All Aspects of the Diabetes Experience

Patients may not immediately raise diabetes-related issues that are viewed as inappropriate to discuss within their culture. For example, patients feeling depressed, anxious, stressed, or shamed may not openly acknowledge these feelings. Patients given diabetes self-management recommendations (e.g., diet, exercise) that conflict with roles and responsibilities in the family also may not readily broach these topics with health care providers. By acknowledging the multiple challenges that patients may encounter, including emotional issues, financial concerns, and family conflicts, we can create a comfortable environment in which to discuss these difficult issues.

SUMMARY

Diabetes patients' economic, social, and cultural context influences their health care and self-management behaviors. To better assist minority patients with diabetes care, we need to think outside of our own medical and cultural environment and step into the environment of our patients. By eliciting our patients' understanding of diabetes, examining the role that family and support systems play in diabetes care, learning the health and illness orientation they embrace, and creating a collaborative relationship of trust and open communication, we can improve diabetes education and care for minority patients.

BIBLIOGRAPHY

Anderson RM, Funnell MM, Arnold MS, Barr PA, Edwards GJ, Fitzgerald JT: Assessing the cultural relevance of an education program for urban African Americans with diabetes. *Diabetes Educ* 26:280–289, 2000

Anderson RM, Herman WH, Davis JM, Freedman RP, Funnell MM, Neighbors HW: Barriers to improving diabetes care for blacks (Editorial). *Diabetes Care* 14:605–609, 1991

Barroso J, McMillan S, Casey L, Gibson W, Kaminski G, Meyer J: Comparison between African-American and white women in their beliefs about breast cancer and their locus of control. *Cancer Nurs* 23:268–276, 2000

Bautista-Martinez S, Aguilar-Salinas CA, Lerman I, Velasco ML, Caste llanos R, Zenteno E, et al.: Diabetes knowledge and its determinants in a Mexican population. *Diabetes Educ* 25:374–381, 1999

Hennessy C, John R, Anderson L: Diabetes education needs of family members caring for American Indian elders. *Diabetes Educ* 5:747–754, 1999

Kleinman A, Eisenberg L, Good B: Culture, illness, and care: clinical lessons from anthropologic and cross-cultural research. *Ann Intern Med* 88:251–258, 1978

Tervalon M, Murray-Garcia J: Cultural humility versus cultural competence: a critical distinction in defining physician training outcomes in multicultural education. *J Health Care Poor Underserved* 9:117–125, 1998

Tripp-Reimer T, Choi E, Skemp Kelley L, Enslein JC: Cultural barriers to care: inverting the problem. *Diabetes Spectrum* 14:13–22, 2001

Wang CY, Abbott L, Goodbody AK, Hui WT, Rausch C: Development of a community-based diabetes management program for Pacific Islanders. *Diabetes Educ* 25:738–746, 1999

Weller SC, Baer RD, Pachter LM, Trotter RT, Glazer M, Garcia de Alba Garcia JE, Klein RE: Latino beliefs about diabetes. *Diabetes Care* 22:722–728, 1999

Robin Nwankwo, MPH, RD, CDE, is a Project Manager at the Michigan Diabetes Research and Training Center at the University of Michigan Medical School in Ann Arbor, MI. Tricia S. Tang, PhD, is an Assistant Professor of Medical Education and the Director of the Sociocultural Medicine Program at the University of Michigan Medical School in Ann Arbor, MI.

Two

Facilitating Self-Care Behaviors

To manage diabetes effectively, people have to follow through on many different kinds of activities every day. They have to eat carefully, stay active, control their weight, not smoke, monitor their blood glucose, and, if they take diabetes medications, recognize, prevent, and treat hypoglycemia as well. Each of these activities is demanding for most people.

In the first chapter of this part, Glasgow discusses the use of interactive technology (IT) to make diabetes self-care behaviors easier for people to maintain. Recent years have seen a dramatic increase in the application of IT to diabetes care, and Glasgow describes some of these developments and offers practical guidance for applying these technologies in clinical practice.

Effective diabetes management requires two kinds of skills: *1)* skill in specific diabetes self-care tasks, such as counting carbohydrates or monitoring blood glucose, and *2)* skill in coping with the demands of applying self-care skills in the context of daily life, where there are often other pressures. In their chapter, Rubin and Peyrot offer suggestions for helping patients develop diabetes-specific coping skills, focusing on the patient's role as the primary provider of diabetes care and how clinicians can help patients make decisions more wisely.

Successfully managing the dietary demands and restrictions of life with diabetes is almost certainly the most common obstacle to effective self-management. In their chapter, Schlundt, Pichert, Gregory, and Davis offer recommendations for an individualized, patient-centered approach to dietary management that integrates ethnic and cultural as well as individual considerations. The authors provide a comprehensive guide to assessing lifestyle and diet and to effective behavioral interventions in this critical area of self-care.

Exercise is another area of self-management that is problematic for many people. Marrero and Sizemore discuss the benefits of regular activity for people with diabetes. They also offer guidelines for helping patients choose the right activity program and for helping patients maintain their motivation to be active. In addition, the authors provide information on risks and recommendations for helping people with complications stay active.

Wing reminds us that weight loss is a key component in the management of obese people who have type 2 diabetes and that avoiding or treating weight gain is important for people with type 1 diabetes as well. Most clinicians have had limited success when trying to help patients with diabetes lose weight; some clinicians have even given up trying. Wing's chapter provides information and strategies to help clinicians and patients see that it is possible to lose weight.

Haire-Joshu discusses the often underappreciated issue of smoking and diabetes. She points out that the prevalence of smoking among adults with diabetes, who are already at a three- to fourfold increased risk for cardiovascular disease, is the same as that in the general population and that the rate of smoking cessation is lower among people with diabetes. The author offers a set of practical guidelines for encouraging patients with diabetes to stop smoking.

Intensive treatment decreases the risk of long-term diabetes complications, but it can also increase the risk of hypoglycemia, including severe hypoglycemia. In their chapter, Gonder-Frederick, Cox, and Clarke provide us with information and techniques to help patients understand, recognize, and cope more effectively with hypoglycemia. Based on their research, the authors developed an intervention called blood glucose awareness training, which has been shown to increase an individual's ability to recognize, avoid, and treat hypoglycemia.

5

Using Interactive Technology in Diabetes Self-Management

RUSSELL E. GLASGOW, PhD

Managing diabetes successfully can be one of life's most challenging tasks. It is the rare individual who manages key lifestyle tasks, such as healthy eating or regular physical activity, perfectly. Even more challenging is combining these tasks with the multitude of other tasks in the diabetes regimen. Data on the staggering health care costs associated with diabetes complications and evidence from the Diabetes Control and Complications Trial and other trials show that tight blood glucose control and diabetes self-management can reduce many of these costly complications. In addition, information systems and self-management are hallmarks of virtually all successful diabetes disease management programs. Such findings make it imperative that patients are helped to self-manage their disease. All too often, however, the difficulty of coping with the demands of the diabetes regimen can overwhelm both patients and clinicians. This chapter provides a framework and practical suggestions for facilitating diabetes self-management and for integrating interactive technology (IT) into this sequence. IT includes various electronic aids to self-management, such as CD-ROM or Internet-based programs, portable computer applications, and automated telephone calls.

ASSESS SELF-MANAGEMENT INFLUENCES, TASKS, AND CONSEQUENCES

Figure 5.1 is intended to help clinicians better understand key self-management issues, set priorities for change efforts, and identify effective intervention strategies. Factors influencing diabetes self-management are shown on the left side of the figure. These factors are arranged in concentric circles based on their proximity to the patient. Note that there are multiple levels of influence that combine to determine self-management. An important implication of this model is that effective self-management is not achieved simply by providing patients with knowledge, but by changing how patients interact with their social environment as well.

The center of the figure represents several different tasks of the diabetes regimen. These tasks are listed separately to illustrate that there is usually little relationship between the extent to which a patient follows one aspect of the regimen and his or her level of self-care in other areas. Stated differently: there are few uniformly good or bad compliers. Most patients show variability in the extent to which they follow different regimen recommendations. It is important to assess the degree of self-management in each area (and not to overwhelm the patient with trying to change everything at once [see Chapter 21]).

Finally, the consequences of self-management, including glycemic control, health outcomes, quality of life, and medical care utilization are shown on the right side of the figure. Self-management and diabetes control are not the same: self-management is one of the multiple determinants of health outcomes (along with genetics, regimen prescriptions, and other factors). A patient's level of self-care cannot be judged from his or her glycated hemoglobin A1C level. For example, a poor medication program may negate or cancel out the benefit of excellent self-management, and vice versa.

The main point of Figure 5.1 is the importance of personalizing the aspect(s) of self-management that a patient needs to target and determining which sets of influences are most relevant or possible to change at a given time (see Chapter 6). The figure also helps us to appreciate the complexity and difficulty of diabetes self-management and demonstrates the inappropriateness of dichotomizing patients into good and bad compliers.

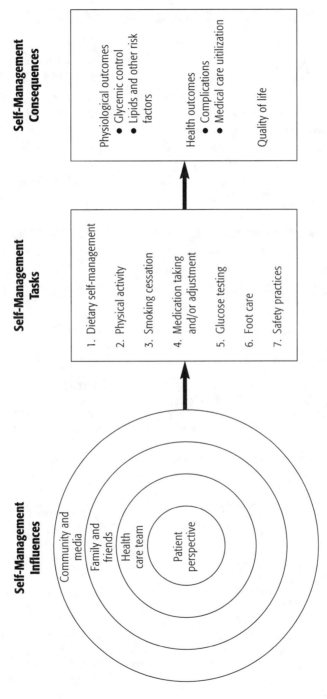

FIGURE 5.1 Diabetes self-management influences, tasks, and consequences.

USE ASSESSMENT AND INTERVENTION STRATEGIES

Although there are times when a comprehensive approach to self-management is optimal (e.g., upon initial diagnosis, when initiating intensive therapy with a multidisciplinary team), at most visits, clinicians have neither the time nor the resources to focus on several different behavioral issues. Also, patients will have greater success if they focus on one or two behaviors between visits.

Table 5.1 and the discussion below provide practical recommendations for a sequence of events that can be accomplished during office visits related to each level of influence on diabetes self-management pictured in Figure 5.1. Also discussed are ways that IT can be used to facilitate each step in this sequence.

Self-management is best thought of as an ongoing series of interactive activities. Figure 5.2 shows how each step in the series leads up to and provides information to use during the later steps. These activities can be performed perfectly well by office staff using open-ended ques-

TABLE 5.1 Self-Management Assessment and Intervention Guidelines

Patient factors
- Assess the degree to which the patient believes that diabetes is serious and that what he or she does to manage it makes a difference.
- Provide personalized feedback on specific effects of diabetes on the patient's health (e.g., "Did you know that diabetes is one of the major risk factors for developing heart disease?").
- Educate the patient on the potential benefits of specific self-management behaviors (e.g., "Regular physical activity helps diabetes control by. . .").

Health care team issues
- Reinforce the same patient goal(s) at a given visit.
- Note in the patient's chart the self-management issues to be followed up on at the next contact.
- Provide follow-up support via phone calls and reviewing goals at subsequent visits.

Social environment
- Assess the patient's barriers to self-management goals (e.g., "Ms. Jones, what things might interfere with you when following the blood glucose testing plan we developed today?").
- Help the patient enlist resources to deal with the barriers you have identified (e.g., "Are you aware of the diabetes support group at the hospital? I think that you might find it quite helpful to talk to others who are dealing with many of the same issues.").

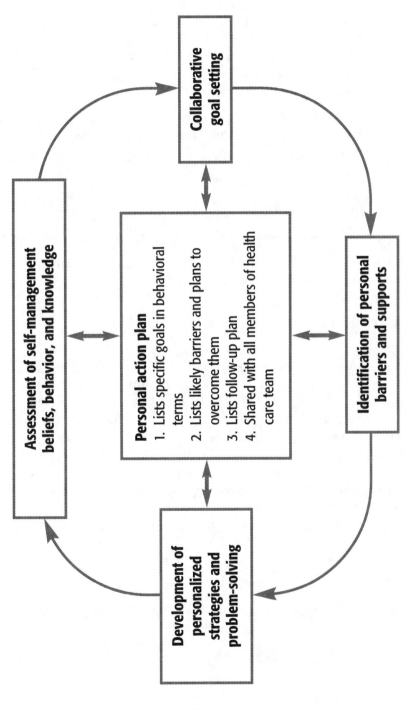

FIGURE 5.2 Behavioral principles expressed as self-management action steps.

tions or paper and pencil, but can also be made more efficient and focused through the use of IT. Using computers or similar devices to ask questions, process information, or provide personally tailored self-management messages or plans can free up the clinician for other important tasks and help guide patient education interactions.

Assessment and Feedback on Self-Management–Related Issues

The first step is to assess what patients are currently doing in the various self-management areas shown in Figure 5.1 and to evaluate their beliefs about the effectiveness of different activities and their willingness to change. Nonjudgmental feedback should be provided regarding how current levels of self-management compare with recommendations and how self-management activities relate to health outcomes. IT can be useful in administering, instantly scoring, and providing visual or multimodal feedback on these issues.

Setting Collaborative Goals

Getting agreement on specific self-management goals is likely the most important aspect of the self-management process. It is usually best to focus on one or two goals for the next visit rather than attempting to change too much at once. These goals should be important to the patient (rather than being what the health care professional considers most important), achievable, and recorded on the action plan (see Chapter 1). In setting goals, the implications for the patient's quality of life should be considered, and it is critical that all members of the health care team reinforce the importance of the goal(s) selected. Most ITs are currently limited in their ability to help patients set individualized goals, but can help start this process by providing a menu of options to consider.

Identifying Barriers and Supports

Integrating self-management plans into the patient's social environment begins with assessment of the anticipated barriers to and availability of resources to support the agreed-upon self-management goals. This can be done by either open-ended questions about what will be likely to interfere with the self-management goal(s) or through an IT or paper and pencil–administered barriers checklist. Both family and community support resources should be enlisted to facilitate long-term success. Examples of community supports include free or low-cost activities (e.g., American Diabetes Association meetings, hospital wellness programs, newsletters, mall walking, or support groups) that can extend the motivation patients receive during office visits.

Problem-Solving

The next step involves working with the patient to identify personally relevant coping strategies to overcome the key barriers identified. Resist the urge to solve problems for the patient. Instead, elicit potential solutions from the patient. Experience suggests that having two or more solutions to a given barrier is advantageous, since no one strategy is likely to work in all situations. A useful procedure to check the adequacy of goal-barrier solution pairings is to have patients rate their confidence on a 10-point scale as to whether they will be able to accomplish their goal(s) between now and their next clinic visit. IT can be useful in getting the brainstorming process started to generate creative strategies but is currently limited in dealing with open-ended responses. IT can be used, for example, to generate a list of possible action strategies that have been successful for previous patients faced with similar barriers. These strategies can then be discussed and patients can select or modify ones that are best for them (see Chapter 6).

Follow-Up Support

A critical but frequently missed step for self-management success is some type of follow-up contact between office visits. Often, just a brief telephone conversation can serve to answer questions, help patients adjust self-management plans, and reinforce their progress. Recent research demonstrates that automated telephone calls to check on patient progress, with back-up by a live staff member, is a widely accepted and effective application of IT for diabetes management. Such calls can use the voice of a familiar office staff member and have been found effective in improving blood glucose monitoring and glycemic control.

Action Plan

As shown in the center of Figure 5.2 and illustrated with the example in Figure 5.3, the action plan serves as a way to integrate and provide a written record of the self-management process. It is important that both the patient and the health care team receive a copy of the action plan, which can then be used at future contacts to guide a brief version of the cycle of iterative activities in Figure 5.2, focusing on changes since the last visit with the patient.

EXAMPLE OF A BRIEF OFFICE-BASED IT-ASSISTED SELF-MANAGEMENT PROGRAM

Our research team has conducted evaluations of several self-management programs assisted by IT. The program described below is designed to be conducted during regular office visits. Through the use of focused assessment instruments and computer technology, we conduct a highly personalized intervention that addresses each of the self-management issues discussed above. This intervention requires only 20 min of additional time from the patient (and nurse or dietitian) and no additional time from the physician. The following description relies on CD-ROM technology. However, these same issues can be addressed almost as efficiently face-to-face or by telephone or mail contacts.

Through the use of touch-screen computerized assessment, we identify specific dietary self-management behaviors leading to high–saturated fat intake. The patient perspective is addressed through assessment of patient beliefs about the seriousness of diabetes and the importance of dietary management. Patients are allowed a choice of areas to address and select a specific goal to work toward. Social-environmental influences (e.g., family members eating foods not consistent with the patient's dietary plan in front of the patient) are addressed by touch-screen assessment of perceived barriers to low-fat eating.

Patient/health care team interactions are facilitated by a computer-generated action plan that summarizes key self-management issues for the patient (Figure 5.3) and by a separate one-page computer printout that summarizes patient goals, barriers, self-management behaviors, and laboratory results for the provider (Figure 5.4). The physician is asked to provide only a brief message about the importance

My Healthy Eating Plan and Reference Guide

My action: *Eat less saturated fats*

Barriers to my action and strategies to overcome barriers:

Barrier 1: I eat out a lot so it's hard to control ingredients and/or portion sizes.

Strategy 1: Choose low-fat condiments to season foods. Try chili peppers, mustard, soy sauce (low sodium), Tabasco sauce, lemon juice, vinegar, salsa, horseradish, and low-calorie salad dressings.

Strategy 2: Skip the bread and butter at the beginning of the meal. Usually, the meal will have plenty of carbohydrates and calories. To assure you are not starving by the time you are seated, eat an apple or a cup of vegetable soup before you go out to eat.

Barrier 2: My family wants high-fat foods and hates fruits and vegetables.

Strategy 1: Don't deprive your family of their favorites; instead, substitute lower-fat ingredients. Grill or broil instead of frying, or use a non-stick pan or nonfat cooking spray. Try baked potatoes with lemon juice instead of butter, cottage cheese instead of sour cream, and instant pudding made with skim milk.

Strategy 2: Wean your family from their fatty foods one step at a time. Switch from whole milk to 2%, to 1%, and then to skim. Switch from whole-fat cheese to partial skim cheese.

Strategy 3: Tell your family that your doctor recommends a healthier diet. Involve them in how to do that. Because people are less likely to resist their own ideas, ask your family for ideas on how to make family meals lower in fat and higher in fruit and vegetables, to help you live a longer, healthier life.

Other barriers, strategies, or notes:

_____

_____

_____

_____

_____

_____

_____

_____

_____

FIGURE 5.3 Patient healthy eating plan and reference guide.

Diabetes Health Connection

Report for Mr. Joe Martinez   *3 August 2001*

GOAL:	ACTION for next 3 months	KEY BARRIERS that interfere with action	STRETEGIES to overcome barriers
Improve Diet	Eat less saturated fat	I eat out a lot; it's hard to control ingredients and/or portions.	• Choose low-fat condiments to season foods. • Skip the bread and butter at the beginning of the meal.
		My family wants high-fat food; hates fruits and vegetables.	• Don't deprive your family of their favorites; instead, substitute lower-fat ingredients. • Wean your family from their fatty foods one at a time.
Increase Physical Activity	Walk for 15 min three times per week	I don't have time.	• Schedule your exercise like you would an important appointment or meeting. • Break up your activity into two or three mini-sessions.
	Bike for 30 min two times per week	The weather prevents me from exercising.	• Ask your local librarian about exercise videos or books to check out. • Try walking at a local mall, which might even open early for mall walkers.

HOW YOUR OFFICE CAN HELP MR. MARTINEZ ACHIEVE THESE GOALS:

1. Ask how the Diabetes Health Connection is going and state that you are glad he is participating.

2. Reinforce importance of healthy eating and regular exercise.

3. Ask how you and your office staff can help support his Diabetes Health Connection plans.

Most recent lab results (assayed ___ / ___ / ___):

Glycated hemoglobin A1C: _____

(normal values from UCHS lab are 4.0–6.0%)

Lipid values: Total cholesterol: _____   LDL: _____

(recommended values are <200 total and <100 LDL.)

Notes: _____

_____

_____

FIGURE 5.4 Diabetes Health Connection provider summary. UCHS, University of Colorado Health Sciences Center.

of self-management and ask the patient to meet with a nurse or health educator to review his or her personalized plan immediately after the physician examination.

The 10- to 20-min self-management session focuses on clarifying any questions the patient has about his or her action plan and making any necessary modifications to goals, barriers, or strategies. To bridge the time until the next quarterly office visit, two brief follow-up phone calls are made to reinforce the patient's progress and help resolve any difficulties.

CONCLUSION

The intervention described above makes substantial use of video and computer technology. Even more sophisticated and efficient IT will be available in the near future with the advent of computerized medical records, automatic provider prompts, and wireless applications. The primary point is not the technology involved—paper and pencil versions of the instruments could be completed by the patient in the waiting room—but rather that a highly personalized, patient-centered intervention can be conducted in a brief period of time. Although there is still a "digital divide" in which minority and lower socioeconomic groups have less access to IT (and especially to high-speed connections), this gap is closing, and several innovative projects have focused on providing IT-assisted health promotion services to such populations.

Key features of the medical office-based intervention approach described in this chapter are that it *1)* addresses the multiple levels of influence on diabetes self-management shown in Figure 5.1 and *2)* incorporates many of the recommended practices in Table 5.1 and Figure 5.2. Probably the single most important thing is that a realistic goal is generated by and makes sense to the patient and is repeatedly reinforced by all members of the health care team.

ACKNOWLEDGMENTS

Preparation of this chapter was supported by grant 3DK RO135524 from the National Institute of Diabetes and Digestive and Kidney Diseases and grant R18 HS10123 from the Agency for Healthcare Research and Quality.

BIBLIOGRAPHY

Anderson LA, Jenkins CM: Educational innovations in diabetes: where are we now? *Diabetes Spectrum* 7:89–124, 1994

Clement S: Diabetes self-management education. *Diabetes Care* 18:1204–1214, 1995

Glasgow RE, Bull SS: Making a difference with interactive technology. *Diabetes Spectrum* 14:99–106, 2001

Glasgow RE, Eakin EG: Medical office-based interventions. In *Psychology in Diabetes Care*. Snoek FJ, Skinner TC, Eds. New York, Wiley, 2000, p. 141–168

Glasgow RE, La Chance P, Toobert DJ, Brown J, Hampson SE, Riddle MC: Long term effects and costs of brief behavioral dietary intervention for patients with diabetes delivered from the medical office. *Patient Educ Couns* 32:175–184, 1997

Litzelman DK, Slemenda CW, Langefeld CD, Hays LM, Welch MA, Bild DE, Ford ES, Vinicor F: Reduction of lower extremity clinical abnormalities in patients with non-insulin-dependent diabetes mellitus: a randomized, controlled trial. *Ann Intern Med* 119:36–41, 1993

Piette JD: Enhancing support via interactive technologies. *Current Diabetes Reports.* In press

Piette JD, Weinberger M, McPhee SJ: The effect of automated calls with telephone nurse follow-up on patient-centered outcomes of diabetes care (a randomized controlled trial). *Med Care* 38:218–230, 2000

Raymond M: *The Human Side of Diabetes: Beyond Doctors, Diets and Drugs.* Chicago, Noble Press, 1992

Russell E. Glasgow, PhD, is a Senior Scientist at the AMC Cancer Research Center in Denver, CO.

6

Helping Patients Develop Diabetes Coping Skills

RICHARD R. RUBIN, PHD, CDE,
AND MARK PEYROT, PHD

Living with diabetes presents countless challenges, from the mundane to the monumental. People who have diabetes must continually pay attention to their treatment regimen, which involves essentially everything they do—eating, sleeping, and physical activity. Many must also take medication to keep their blood glucose levels as close to normal as possible, and all should monitor their glucose levels regularly in an effort to achieve this goal. The diabetes self-care regimen is complex, unremitting, and unpleasant. Yet, in spite of these demands, following the regimen does not guarantee that blood glucose levels will be normal or that complications will be completely avoided. Most people with diabetes walk the line between hyperglycemia and the attendant fear of chronic diabetes complications, and hypoglycemia and the fear of acute complications. They may in fact experience potentially devastating complications.

People who have diabetes frequently say they feel frustrated, fed up, overwhelmed, or burned-out (see Chapters 20 and 21). Or they may report feeling chronically angry, guilty, or fearful. Whereas other aspects of life certainly contribute to this distress, the problems of living with diabetes are also a factor. Distress created by living with diabetes can trigger a negative cascade involving diminished motivation, less active self-care, higher blood glucose levels, increased risk of complications, and a poorer quality of life.

Coping effectively with the myriad challenges of life with diabetes can activate a positive cascade, leading to enhanced motivation, more active self-care, improved metabolic outcomes, and a better quality of life. The health care provider can help patients build diabetes-specific coping skills. This chapter offers guidelines for this process.

RECOGNIZE THAT THE PATIENT IS IN CONTROL

People who have diabetes make countless decisions every day that directly affect their health. In fact, the cumulative effect of these decisions concerning eating, activity, medication, blood glucose monitoring, and seeking health care far outweighs the impact of the health care provider's much less frequent interventions. Some people make self-care decisions wisely; others may be unaware there are even decisions to make. But for all people with diabetes, these decisions powerfully affect blood glucose control and physical and emotional well-being.

People with diabetes make most of the clinically relevant decisions, and they *control* these decisions as well. This is evident every time a clinician's carefully crafted treatment recommendations goes unheeded. Patients sometimes follow provider recommendations, but this may not reflect either the wisdom of the provider's suggestions or the provider's control over patient choices. Patients follow recommendations when—and only when—these recommendations make sense to them (i.e., the benefit is clear and the burden seems bearable) (see Chapter 1). Diabetes care is driven by patient choices, not by health care provider actions.

Still, health care providers are experts in the clinical management of diabetes, so they play a critical role in helping patients make wise choices. Because of their expertise, health care providers are ideal *consultants* who are seeking to make diabetes management as easy and effective as possible. The provider's goal is to help patients solve diabetes-related problems and develop diabetes coping skills, so they will be better able to solve emerging problems on their own.

START WITH THE PATIENT'S AGENDA

The key to accomplishing this goal is focusing on the problems that concern the patient most. These are the issues patients are most motivated to resolve, and solving these problems builds diabetes problem-solving skills and confidence for addressing other diabetes-related problems. Start with questions like:

- "What concerns you most about your diabetes?"
- "What is the hardest thing for you right now about living with diabetes?"
- "What issues would you like to talk about today?"

Starting with the patient's agenda clarifies and reinforces the diabetes management roles of the patient and the health care provider. The person with diabetes is the chief executive officer (i.e., the person who makes the key decisions) and the chief operating officer (i.e., the person who implements the decisions), whereas the health care provider is the expert consultant (i.e., the person who knows a lot of potentially helpful things). Diabetes management is most effective when the person with diabetes sets the agenda and makes the decisions and the health care provider offers options for action, helping the patient solve specific problems and build generally applicable diabetes coping skills.

HELP PATIENTS TO SPECIFY THEIR PROBLEMS

Helping patients find specific key problems in their lives with diabetes, what we have termed "sticking points" (problems that patients cannot get past), facilitates diabetes-specific coping. These diabetes-related sticking points (like feeling deprived of a cherished treat) can activate the negative cascade of frustration, less active diabetes care, and diminished health and quality of life described earlier. Resolving sticking points can trigger a positive cascade, including enhanced motivation, more active self-care, closer-to-normal blood glucose levels, reduced risk of complications, and better quality of life.

It is important to help patients define these sticking points specifically, because general formulations of problems ("I can't do anything right," "I cannot eat the way I should," or "I cannot lose weight") are overwhelming emotionally and do not provide a basis for identifying solutions (see Chapter 21). To illustrate the benefits of focusing on a specific sticking point, we offer the following example.

A man sought treatment from one of the authors (R.R.R.), stating he was a "bad diabetic" who did "nothing right." A few questions uncovered the man's specific sticking point: no matter what he tried, he could not stop snacking between dinner and bedtime. As a result, the man was up many times each night to urinate (a result of hyperglycemia), and he dragged himself through the next day exhausted, guilty, and discouraged.

Identifying a specific sticking point is often a source of relief for patient and provider alike because it narrows the scope of the problem and provides a focused target for intervention. This man identified several possible ways to curb his evening snacking and was able to avoid excessive snacking several nights each week. This behavior change was a real improvement, and the patient felt revitalized by his success.

Patients often describe their diabetes coping challenges in broad terms; they may say that everything bothers them or that their major difficulty is their diet. With encouragement, almost every person can identify more specific sticking points. We often ask patients to give a specific example of what happens, tell a story of a recent incident, or walk us through the situation step-by-step. We sometimes suggest that patients identify their problem so specifically that we could take a photograph or make a video of it, and this generally helps.

FOCUS ON THE PATIENT'S SUCCESSES

One of the most important and useful set of questions to ask is, "Can you remember a time when the situation went better than usual? How come things worked out so well that time?" There will be times when a situation that can be a problem goes better than usual, and figuring out what helped can be tremendously beneficial. This approach helped with the patient we just described. It turned out that this man occasionally avoided excessive snacking even before he sought treatment for his problem. As we talked about these rare successes, the patient recognized that this happened only when he was thinking about his young grandson. On these occasions, he would unconsciously say to himself, "I want to be alive 15 years from now to see that boy walk across the stage and get his high school diploma." And that did the trick.

Whatever the reason a problem situation goes more smoothly than it usually does (and the reason may be unique to the individual), helping patients figure out what made things work better will help them improve coping skills and self-care. And, by focusing on successes rather than failures, this method will help the patient learn in the most effective possible way.

INVOLVE THE PATIENT'S FAMILIES

Diabetes is a family disease: the demands of diabetes and its management affect everyone who loves, lives with, or cares for a person who has diabetes. And the behavior of those individuals close to the patient affects the patient's self-care. Some patients feel that family and friends ignore their diabetes and do not support their efforts to manage the disease (e.g., "Eat a little cake; a bite won't hurt you," or, "Why do we always have to wait for dinner until after you test your blood?"). Others feel their family and friends go to the opposite extreme, monitoring and criticizing every action that could affect blood glucose levels (e.g., "You know that cookie is not on your diet; are you trying to kill yourself?," or, "You haven't walked in weeks. You'll never control your diabetes that way."). Either reaction—minimizing the demands of diabetes management, or harassment—adds stress to the life of a person with diabetes, generating feelings of anger, guilt, frustration, and isolation. Living with these feelings is bad enough, but these feelings also can compromise self-care, physical well-being, and the quality of a person's most important relationships.

The most appropriate help for a patient with support problems will depend on the specific situation. If family members' lack of support or over-involvement stems from a lack of knowledge or understanding about diabetes and diabetes care, attending diabetes education classes or reading books or magazines that discuss these issues might be helpful. Meeting with the person who has diabetes and his or her family might also facilitate more constructive interaction and communication (see Chapter 19). If the patient or family members do not choose to meet in this setting, asking the patient some basic questions may help. The patient should be asked to offer examples of ways family and friends make it easier to manage diabetes, examples of ways they make it harder to manage diabetes, and specific, realistic changes others could make that would help the person feel more supported or less harassed. Counseling the patient in ways to effectively communicate a desire for change will facilitate the process.

SUPPORT DIABETES COPING SKILLS

The goal of working with patients should not only be to help them resolve or cope with their diabetes-related problems; we need to help them develop the skills to deal with such problems on their own. Sometimes this means letting them work out their own solutions to problems, even if the solution seems obvious. One of us (R.R.R.) was taking his teenage son out to dinner after his son had begun using an insulin pump only a few days earlier. The meal was a special occasion, and the young man had talked his father into letting him order anything he wanted. Unfortunately, his predinner blood glucose level was 350 mg/dl. Taking a chance on his son's budding diabetes problem-solving skills and hoping to strengthen them, the father agreed to stick with the agreement on the condition that the young man think really hard about how much insulin he needed to take to cover the meal and that he test his blood 2 and 4 h after dinner. Even after a big dinner, the results of these tests were 220 and 150 mg/dl. The boy explained his success: "I calculated how much carbohydrate was in each thing I ate, and I used the formula I was taught to figure the amount of insulin I needed. I really wanted that food, and I really didn't want to feel sick later, so I worked hard to get the insulin right."

One way to facilitate the development of coping skills is to explain to patients what the problem-solving process is. As you are working to help patients identify their specific sticking points, explain why specificity is important and encourage them to be specific when they are trying to understand the nature of their own problems. Talk about how prior success is the key to future success. Ultimately, your greatest contribution will be in preparing patients to cope with their day-to-day problems without having to wait until they can see you.

HELP BUILD EMOTIONAL STRENGTH

Coping effectively with diabetes requires emotional strength as well as problem-solving skills. We've found that love, optimism, and humor are key elements of emotional strength. Clinicians would do well to foster these qualities in their patients (and themselves as well; see Chapter 3).

When it comes to coping with the stress of life with diabetes, love gives us confidence and motivation and is a powerful source of emotional well-being. Ask your patients if the hassles and aggravations of daily life with diabetes are preventing them and their families from enjoying, appreciating, and loving each other.

Optimism is another bulwark against the stresses and strains of daily life with diabetes. Encourage patients and loved ones to draw upon all sources of optimism. Think of the improvements being made in diabetes care. Think about the positive aspects of diabetes. For example, 40 years ago, a 13-year-old girl became the first person in her family to be diagnosed with diabetes. When the girl asked her mother what having diabetes would mean for them, her mother responded, "It means we will learn to eat better than we have ever eaten before, we will all be healthier than we ever were before, and we will all learn to love each other more than we ever did before."

One of the authors spoke with a 54-year-old man several months after the man was diagnosed with diabetes. The man noted the difficulties he was having adjusting to some aspects of his new regimen, but he quickly added, "It's not all bad. I've started walking in the evenings, and that has been just great. My wife and I head out after dinner at least three nights a week. We walk and talk. We've been married 33 years, and I don't think we've ever felt closer. And that's not all; we've each lost a few pounds and we feel good about that." Dealing with a challenge together can heighten intimacy.

Humor is another wonderful coping strategy. It helps keep things in perspective and protects people from feeling overwhelmed. The essence of humor is taking a bad situation and exaggerating its awfulness to the point it is so ridiculous it becomes funny. Fortunately or unfortunately, life with diabetes presents us with plenty of material for humor. Try to find some humor in patients' daily experiences and see what can be made of it. A woman woke up in the middle of the night in the throes of a hypoglycemic reaction. Her usual antidotes (graham crackers and juice) were not by her bed, and she was too shaky to make it down to the kitchen herself, so she woke her husband. He dragged himself out of bed and staggered groggily down the stairs. As the minutes ticked by, the woman lay in bed waiting and shaking from her reaction. Finally, she started to crawl out of bed to get the food she needed (and to find out what had happened to her husband). When he came staggering back up the stairs, still half asleep and empty handed, the woman cried, "Where is my food?" "Oh no! I ate it myself," the chagrined husband responded. Needless to say, his second trip to the kitchen for food was quicker than the first had been. In a few minutes, the woman's blood glucose level was heading back to normal. At that point, they shared a good laugh about how ridiculous the situation had been and quickly went peacefully and happily back to sleep.

Identifying and discussing any positive diabetes-related experiences can help patients cope better with their diabetes. These experiences are rare for most people, but the fact that they exist at all may have a powerful salutary effect, relieving distress in the moment and enhancing motivation for diabetes care in the long run. Clinicians will be providing a real service if they can help patients and their families to find love, optimism, and humor in their lives with diabetes. And, again, helping them to look for these things on their own is better than waiting until they come to see you.

FIND OTHER RESOURCES TO HELP PATIENTS

There will be times when diabetes is too much for a person to cope with, even with the help and support of a health care team and family. When this is true, try to direct the patient to other resources available in your community. Some people with diabetes benefit from participating in diabetes support groups organized by local hospitals. If the patient is suffering from depression or another psychological disorder, this might mean referral for specialized mental health services by a professional who also knows about diabetes. See the Chapter 22 on depression for criteria to use in deciding if referral to a mental health professional is warranted and for suggestions about making referrals in a way that is helpful and constructive. Getting help can also mean helping the patient and his or her family find a diabetes education program that includes coping skills training. At the Johns Hopkins Diabetes Center, we have developed such a program. The coping skills training component uses the approach described here, developing problem-solving and emotional coping skills. The benefits of this program are wide-ranging, including improvements in emotional well-being, self-care behavior, and glycemic control.

CONCLUSION

Coping effectively with the myriad challenges of life with diabetes can activate a positive cascade, leading to enhanced motivation, more active self-care, improved metabolic outcomes, and a better quality of life. The health care provider can help patients build diabetes-specific coping skills.

BIBLIOGRAPHY

Anderson RM, Funnell M: *The Art of Empowerment: Stories and Strategies for Diabetes Educators.* Alexandria, VA, American Diabetes Association, 2000

Polonsky WH: *Diabetes Burnout: What to Do When You Can't Take It Anymore.* Alexandria, VA, American Diabetes Association, 1999

Rollnick S, Mason P, Butler C: *Health Behavior Change: A Guide for Practitioners.* London, Churchill Livingstone, 1999

Rubin RR: Facilitating self-care in people with diabetes. *Diabetes Spectrum* 14:55–57, 2001

Rubin RR, Biermann J, Toohey B: *Psyching Out Diabetes.* 3rd ed. Los Angeles, CA, Lowell House, 1999

Rubin RR, Peyrot M: Psychological issues and treatments for people with diabetes. *J Clin Psychol* 57:457–478, 2001

Rubin RR, Peyrot M, Saudek CD: Differential effect of diabetes education on self-regulation and lifestyle behaviors. *Diabetes Care* 14:335–338, 1991

Rubin RR, Peyrot M, Saudek CD: The effect of a diabetes education program incorporating coping skills training on emotional well-being and diabetes self-efficacy. *Diabetes Educ* 19:210–214, 1993

Richard R. Rubin, PhD, CDE, is an Associate Professor of Medicine and Pediatrics at The Johns Hopkins University School of Medicine in Baltimore, MD. Mark Peyrot, PhD, is Chair of the Department of Sociology and the Director of the Center for Social and Community Research at Loyola College in Baltimore, MD.

7

Eating and Diabetes: A Patient-Centered Approach

DAVID G. SCHLUNDT, PhD,
JAMES W. PICHERT, PhD,
BECKY GREGORY, MS, RD, LDN, CDE, AND
DIANNE DAVIS, RD, LDN, CDE

Nutrition is a major component of the management of type 1 and type 2 diabetes. Unfortunately, many health care professionals feel discouraged about their ability to help patients make and maintain changes in eating behavior (see Chapter 3). For many years, the dominant approach was to prescribe a rigid diet. Now, advances in diabetes care and management make other approaches to nutrition therapy possible. In this chapter, we describe an approach that we call "patient-centered diabetes care."

WHAT IS PATIENT-CENTERED DIABETES CARE?

The goals of nutrition therapy in diabetes are as follows: *1*) maintaining near-normal blood glucose levels, *2*) achieving optimum serum lipid levels, *3*) providing adequate calories for growth and/or maintenance of a reasonable body weight, *4*) preventing acute and chronic complications of diabetes, and *5*) promoting wellness through optimal nutrition. To better meet these goals, the American Diabetes Association has published guidelines for the nutrition management of diabetes. The guidelines call for an individualized, patient-centered approach that integrates nutrition therapy into the individual's lifestyle—an approach that is sensitive to ethnic, cultural, and individual differences.

Instead of the traditional approach of prescribing specific numbers or percentages of calories, carbohydrates, protein, and fats, patient-centered nutrition management involves:

- Assessing the patient's current eating habits, insulin or medication use, and patterns of exercise and physical activity
- Starting with current lifestyle and negotiating a medical management plan that will achieve good control with an acceptable degree of lifestyle change
- Sharing realistic expectations concerning the difficulty of meeting glucose targets in everyday situations
- Sustaining life-long self-management practices that minimize complications while maximizing quality of life
- Teaching behavioral strategies that help patients to achieve and sustain successes in daily life

ASSESS EATING PATTERNS AND LIFESTYLE

Before a plan can be negotiated, the provider must understand the patient's current eating habits: the who, what, when, where, why, and how often of what each patient eats. Foods do not just fill our stomachs, and they are much more than blends of micronutrients and macronutrients. Foods have cultural, interpersonal, and emotional meanings that must be understood to negotiate a realistic plan of diabetes self-management.

Assessment involves a combination of interview questions, diaries, and structured questionnaires. Questionnaires can emphasize nutritional information, such as a food frequency questionnaire, or can focus on behaviors or on how people respond to challenging situations. A diet diary in which patients record foods, amounts, and the circumstances surrounding their eating can also be a useful assessment tool. A food diary can provide valuable information about the blood glucose response to difficult foods such as high-fat foods or alcohol. Diaries can also be used to gather information about problem situations such as holiday meals or eating away from home. The provider's goal is to learn about current eating habits, what strengths an individual has, and where weaknesses and problems exist.

Table 7.1 presents common lifestyle influences on dietary adherence. Each entry represents a type of everyday situation that makes adherence difficult and suggests interview questions to use during an assessment.

BUILD MEDICAL MANAGEMENT AROUND LIFESTYLE

Patient-centered nutrition and medical management in diabetes involves the following key elements:

Glucose monitoring and target ranges. Managing blood glucose requires:

- Frequent and well-timed feedback on current glucose levels
- An agreeable schedule for blood glucose self-monitoring
- Negotiated blood glucose target ranges; target ranges depend on the patient's desired degree of control, risk for hypoglycemia, commitment to preventing complications, and resources and abilities
- Access to monitoring equipment and supplies and the resources to pay for them
- Training in the appropriate use of equipment

Quantifying food intake. To regulate blood glucose, patients need to learn to use a method for quantifying their food intake. Commonly used strategies include exchange groups, carbohydrate gram counting, and the food guide pyramid. Patients with type 2 diabetes who want to lose weight may also benefit from learning to count fat grams and/or calories, whereas patients with lipid problems may need to monitor carbohydrates and monounsaturated fats. The specific method should reflect the patient's goals, abilities, and preferences and should be used to help patients make intelligent self-management decisions (see Chapter 1).

Making adjustments in food, medication, and activity. When a person has a stable and routine lifestyle, it may be possible to take the same insulin or oral medication, eat the same amount of food, and engage in consistent physical activity, minimizing the need for adjustments. Most patients, however, will need to learn how to adjust food and activity to compensate for hyperglycemia and hypoglycemia. Patients who take

TABLE 7.1 **Assessing Lifestyle and Diet**

Type of problem	Description	Interview questions
Negative emotions	The patient overeats to cope with stress and negative feelings.	Are there any situations in your life that are currently causing you a lot of stress? Do you eat differently when you feel upset, depressed, or stressed?
Resisting temptation	Foods, cues, and cravings tempt the patient to eat inappropriate foods.	What foods or situations trigger cravings? What foods or situations tempt you to eat inappropriately?
Eating out	Eating away from home (e.g., restaurants) makes it hard for the patient to control what and how much he or she eats.	How do the amounts or kinds of foods you eat differ when you eat away from home or at a restaurant?
Feeling deprived	The patient feels deprived because he or she cannot eat foods he or she enjoys and is tempted to give up and give in.	How often do you feel like giving up on taking good care of your diabetes because it keeps you from eating the way you enjoy? What foods do you feel you should give up eating?
Time pressure	The many demands on the patient's time makes healthy eating difficult.	What kinds of social, family, or job pressures make it hard for you to find the time to eat the way you want to?
Tempted to relapse	The patient feels discouraged or like a failure and considers no longer trying to eat right.	How often do you feel so discouraged about your eating plan that you want to just give up? Do you see your current plan as rigid or flexible?
Planning	A hectic schedule makes it hard for the patient to plan what and when to eat.	How difficult is it for you to plan when, where, and what you will eat?
Competing priorities	The patient has many responsibilities and obligations (e.g., family and job) that interfere with the ability to make healthy food choices.	What important priorities in your life get in the way of making healthy food choices? Do you sometimes feel like you have to choose between good diabetes care and other important life goals?

Social events	The patient overeats at parties, holidays, special occasions, and other social events that involve food.	How do the amounts or kinds of food you eat differ when you eat at parties or social events?
Family support	The patient's family does not support healthy food choices.	Describe the things your family does to support or hinder your efforts to eat the way you want to.
Food refusal	When an inappropriate food is offered, the patient finds it hard to refuse.	How hard is it for you to refuse food when someone offers it to you?
Friends' support	The patient's friends do not support healthy food choices.	Describe the things your friends do to support or hinder your efforts to eat the way you want to.
All-or-nothing thinking	The patient sees himself or herself and the world in black-and-white terms and alternates between being in and out of control of eating.	How do you react when you are unable to achieve an important goal or if you are unable to stick to a plan? Are there times when you alternate between being in control and out of control?

Adapted from Schlundt DG, Rea MR, Kline SS, Pichert JW: Situational obstacles to dietary adherence for adults with diabetes. *J Am Diet Assoc* 94:874–876, 1994.

insulin can learn to adjust insulin and use sliding scales, giving them additional flexibility in responding to low and high blood glucose values.

Problem-solving: the ongoing process of monitoring and adjusting. Table 7.1 identifies many everyday situations in which decisions have to be made and implemented to keep blood glucose in the target range. Patient-centered diabetes management includes helping people learn how to anticipate, prevent, and solve daily problems as they arise (see Chapter 6). The process is one of regular blood glucose monitoring and adjusting food, insulin, activity, or thinking to cope with each challenging situation.

Patient choice and flexibility in goals. No single approach to nutrition management will work for everyone. Patients must participate in selecting their goals and strategies. Some will prefer highly structured approaches and a well-defined meal plan. Others will prefer the flexibility of adjusting insulin to match carbohydrate consumption. In a patient-centered approach, the range of options is discussed and a plan is tailored to the individual's needs and preferences.

In general, the same self-management principles for people on insulin apply to patients with type 2 diabetes who are not using insulin. Individuals with type 2 diabetes who do not take insulin will have to learn to adjust food intake and physical activity to achieve blood glucose goals. Besides strategies for keeping blood glucose in a target range, the management of type 2 diabetes may include efforts to lose weight, reduce fat intake, consume a moderate carbohydrate intake, optimally space meal times, and/or increase exercise. Losing modest amounts of weight and increasing physical activity involve individually negotiated goals, flexibility in how to achieve those goals, and ability to solve problems as they arise. Because long-term maintenance of weight loss is difficult, individualized goals, flexibility, and ongoing problem-solving are critical for lasting success (see Chapter 9).

HELP PATIENTS BE REALISTIC

Patient-centered diabetes management requires realistic expectations.

Compromise is to be expected. Almost everyone will need to make some lifestyle changes. People whose lifestyles are erratic, haphazard, high-stress, or in some way incompatible with even the most flexible of diabetes management plans will have to compromise. Both patient and provider need to compromise to negotiate a workable self-management plan.

Skills are learned gradually. Diabetes self-management requires many skills such as blood glucose self-monitoring, sliding insulin scales, counting carbohydrate grams, and being more assertive with family members. People do need time to master these skills, along with generous helpings of feedback, encouragement, and patience.

Slips and relapses are common. Changes in lifestyle do not automatically become permanent, and it is common for patients to fall short of their goals from time to time. The key to long-term success is to learn to cope effectively with these periodic lapses in self-management and to avoid allowing a slip to turn into a full-blown relapse. Long-term success involves monitoring, adjusting, and problem-solving in ever-changing circumstances that challenge an individual's ability to keep blood glucose in the target range or to take the steps needed to prevent complications. Teach patients to expect difficulty, plan ahead for it, and seek support when trouble occurs. Perfect performance in all situations is unrealistic (see Chapter 21).

Problems will not go away if you ignore them. Difficulties, relapses, and stressful episodes occur in everyone's life. Ignoring these problems will not make them go away. Many patients, however, use the strategy of denial when faced with difficulties. Sometimes, a provider's first task is to help a patient admit that there is a problem. Only then is it possible to negotiate goals, create plans, and begin to work toward solutions (see Chapter 20).

The key to realistic expectations is reasonable goals. Frequent contact and fostering honest and open communication facilitates long-term success. Accept problems when they occur and work to solve them. Avoid blaming, scolding, and scaring people. These negative strategies rarely, if ever, work. Instead, ask the patient, "What are you willing and able to do to get your blood sugar under better control?"

FACILITATE DIETARY SELF-MANAGEMENT

Diet instruction should *1)* facilitate good diabetes control and *2)* foster wellness through healthy eating habits. Advances in blood glucose self-monitoring, types of insulin, and insulin delivery regimens and new oral medications make it unnecessary for people to be forced to follow a rigid diet. Instead of emphasizing diets, the focus is on appropriate self-management. Ultimately, each person is responsible for what he or she eats and drinks and for the health outcomes resulting from these choices. Self-management means a person learns to modify choices to meet short-term and long-term health goals.

The primary concern for patients with type 2 diabetes is achieving adequate blood glucose control. However, patients with type 2 diabetes are at higher risk for heart disease than the general population because of concurrent problems with high blood pressure, obesity, and hyperlipidemia. Dietary self-management, therefore, may also mean learning to make food and beverage choices that lower the risk of heart disease. Success in reducing heart disease risk involves knowledge, motivation, skill, and persistence. The patient must know what foods to emphasize and which to limit. Because many other goals and priorities compete with healthy eating for a person's time and attention, a strong commitment to healthy eating is required. Skills such as reading food labels, counting fat grams, ordering healthy meals in restaurants, modifying recipes, or overcoming long-standing problems with binge eating may have to be mastered. Prevention of heart disease is a lifelong process, and persistence is necessary to overcome a constant stream of situations that challenge the patient's knowledge, skill, and commitment to healthy eating.

Flexibility, realistic goals, and ongoing support are more important than factual education in helping people master dietary self-management. Each person is different, each faces unique challenges, and each proceeds at his or her own pace toward the long-term goals of good diabetes care.

KEEP IN MIND DIETARY RULES OF THUMB

Consider teaching your patients these five behavioral guidelines for successful dietary self-management:

1. **Be consistent.** The more predictable the timing, composition, and size of meals, the less decision-making and adjustment required. Consistent habits are the basis of a successful plan for diabetes care.
2. **When you can't be consistent, be close.** When eating the usual amount or kinds of food is impossible, choosing similar foods makes for less adjustment and decision-making.

3. **When you aren't close, make adjustments.** Often circumstances lead to deviations in the amount, composition, or timing of meals. On these occasions, problem-solving and decision-making are needed to identify and implement adjustments that will quickly return blood glucose to the target range.
4. **Be prepared, plan ahead.** Many difficulties can be avoided by looking ahead and making plans to be prepared.
5. **Avoid all-or-none thinking.** When deviations, unexpected difficulties, or circumstances requiring problem-solving and adjustment arise, do not view these times as instances of failure. Replace the kind of black-and-white thinking that sees choices as either successes or failures with realistic goals, self-acceptance, and moderation.

There is no one best way to solve dietary self-management problems. In practice, people must be flexible, approaching problems with a hierarchy of strategies ranging from choosing consistent meals to making complex regimen adjustments.

RECOGNIZE THE ROLE OF THE DIABETES TEAM

The goals of improving dietary self-management and building problem-solving skills are impossible to accomplish in a 15-min doctor's visit. Success involves a team approach. Patient-centered team care requires:

- A well-trained team of qualified professionals.
- A case manager for each patient who is responsible for ensuring that the expertise of the other team members is used as needed.
- Open lines of communication between the patient and the team, and among team members.
- A commitment to basing decisions on what will be best for the patient rather than what will be most convenient for the providers.

Implementing patient-centered diabetes care is not easy. Just as patients face many obstacles in achieving good glycemic control, treatment teams will face many obstacles in implementing patient-centered team management, such as third-party reimbursement, distinctions between disciplinary domains of expertise, institutional pressures to see more patients in less time, cultural and economic barriers that separate patient from professional, and the effects of professional stress and burnout (see Chapter 3).

ACKNOWLEDGMENTS

This work was supported by National Institutes of Health Grant P60 DK20593.

BIBLIOGRAPHY

American Diabetes Association: Evidence-based nutrition principles and recommendations for the treatment and prevention of diabetes and related complications (Position Statement). *Diabetes Care* 25:202–212, 2002

American Diabetes Association: Nutrition recommendations and principles for people with diabetes mellitus (Position Statement). *Diabetes Care* 24 (Suppl. 1):S44–S48, 2001

DCCT Research Group: Nutrition interventions for intensive therapy in the Diabetes Control and Complications Trial. *J Am Diet Assoc* 93:768–772, 1993

Gregory RP, Davis DL: Use of carbohydrate counting for meal planning in type I diabetes. *Diabetes Educ* 20:406–409, 1994

Monk A, Barry B, McClain D, Weaver T, Cooper N, Franz M: Practice guidelines for medical nutrition therapy by dietitians for persons with non-insulin-dependent diabetes mellitus. *J Am Diet Assoc* 95:999–1008, 1995

Nutall FQ, Chasuk RM: Nutrition and the management of type 2 diabetes. *J Fam Pract* 47 (Suppl. 5):S45–S53, 1998

Schlundt DG, Rea MR, Kline SS, Pichert JW: Situational obstacles to dietary adherence for adults with diabetes. *J Am Diet Assoc* 94:874–876, 1994

David G. Schlundt, PhD, is an Associate Professor of Psychology at Vanderbilt University in Nashville, TN. James W. Pichert, PhD, is an Associate Professor of Education in Medicine at the Diabetes Research and Training Center at Vanderbilt University School of Medicine, and is Associate Professor of Psychology and Human Development at Peabody College in Nashville, TN. Becky Gregory, MS, RD, LDN, CDE, is a Nutrition Coordinator and Dianne Davis, RD, LDN, CDE, is a Research Dietitian at the Diabetes Research and Training Center at Vanderbilt University School of Medicine in Nashville, TN.

8

Facilitating Physical Activity in People with Diabetes

DAVID G. MARRERO, PhD, AND JILL SIZEMORE, MS

> *Exercise in the days before insulin we regarded as useful, but by no means did we appreciate it as vital in the care of diabetes. . . . We should return to it to help us in the treatment of all of our cases. . . .* (Joslin et al, *Treatment of Diabetes Mellitus*, 1959)

Increasing evidence supports what Joslin observed over 40 years ago: consistent, regular physical activity has many benefits for people with either type 1 or type 2 diabetes. These benefits include weight control, a reduced need for insulin and/or oral hypoglycemic agents, and improved control of glycemia, blood pressure, and blood lipid levels, thereby reducing the risk of complications. Moreover, there is increasing evidence that physical activity can even help prevent diabetes in individuals at increased risk for the disease.

In spite of these benefits, many people with diabetes are not active on a regular basis. Health care providers are often unsure of what constitutes an appropriate exercise regimen for their patients with diabetes, and many people with diabetes, notably those with type 2, are resistant to becoming more active. Still, health care professionals are in a unique position to help patients begin and maintain an effective and safe activity program. In this chapter, we offer several suggestions on how best to accomplish this goal. These suggestions are based on three intuitively simple, yet often neglected, axioms:

1. Promote a program that is intrinsically reinforcing for patients.
2. Recommend a program that is realistic, feasible, and, most importantly, sustainable for patients.

3. Educate patients on how to avoid the potential negative consequences of exercise, particularly those associated specifically with diabetes.

PROMOTE A PROGRAM THAT IS DESIRABLE AND REINFORCING

To help patients adopt programs for increasing physical activity, we need to consider the forces that shape their decisions to do so. Three basic principles of behavior modification apply:

1. **Perceived benefits.** The first and most basic principle is that motivation to begin any new behavior, such as a regular activity program, is grounded in the patient's perception of the benefits of that behavior and the importance of obtaining those benefits. In this regard, what a patient perceives as a benefit may be idiosyncratic. For example, some people may be motivated to increase physical activity to lower the risk of complications, others to control weight, and others to achieve feelings of self-control.

2. **Perceived costs.** The second principle is that a behavior is not likely to be initiated and maintained if the costs associated with the activity outweigh the benefits. Like benefits, costs are often idiosyncratically defined and can include physical, social, or psychological factors, including pain, the threat of hypoglycemia, imposition of additional responsibilities, and fear of failure.

3. **Reinforcement.** The third principle is that reinforcement for initiating and maintaining a behavior is most effective when it is experienced immediately. And in almost all cases, positive reinforcement is more effective than punishment. Thus, reducing the risk of long-term complications may be less effective in reinforcing physical activity than increased fitness, reduced weight, or other more immediate positive outcomes (see Chapter 15).

HELP BUILD THE FOUNDATION FOR MOTIVATION

To begin the process of facilitating motivation for increased activity, help patients identify the potential benefits of exercise that matter most to them. Documented benefits of activity for people with diabetes include the following:

- Health benefits, such as improvements in glucose regulation, weight control, lipid profiles, hypertension, and increased work capacity.
- Social benefits, such as increased interaction with family members and "social others" (i.e., training partners) and participation in organized, community-based activities.
- Psychological benefits—most notably reduced anxiety, depression, and stress and increased feelings of well-being.

In addition to these benefits, it is important to emphasize the following key points:

Physical activity is part of a life-long management program. Patients should not expect to begin exercising at a high intensity. Together, the patient and provider should select a series of goals that are safe, are achievable, and will help the patient develop an effective program over time.

Even modest activity has health benefits. The person with diabetes does not have to become an elite athlete to realize health benefits from physical activity. Research shows that even modest levels of activity, such as brisk walking for 30 min a day, can produce considerable health benefits.

Physical activity can take many forms. For some people, the concept of structured exercise is simply not a pleasant thought. It is important to emphasize that there are simple ways to increase activity levels without following a structured exercise program. For example, use the stairs instead of the elevator or park farther from the store and walk a bit more. In this context, it is also important to note that several small sessions of activity can have the same benefits as one longer session.

People have to learn how to properly exercise, i.e., to be active without discomfort, injury, or added problems with diabetes management. This result will require experimenting with new behaviors, including adjusting the patient's diabetes regimen.

Providers are available as a resource. Health care professionals and others in their communities are there to help patients accomplish these goals.

The best activity plan fits an individual's specific needs. These needs include physical condition, goals, desires, and the availability of time and appropriate support.

Having laid this foundation, clinicians will be ready to help patients select exercise programs that are likely to be sustained over time.

HELP PATIENTS SELECT THE RIGHT EXERCISE PROGRAM

Specific exercise prescriptions help patients successfully increase physical activity. Generic prescriptions, with little or no guidance concerning what to do, how to do it, or how to adjust the diabetes regimen to safely exercise, are rarely helpful. By discussing with patients two simple, related questions, clinicians can help patients design a specific activity prescription that they are likely to enjoy (see Chapter 6). These questions are:

What are your goals for exercise? Identifying patients' exercise goals helps identify the activities most likely to achieve these goals. Remember, what patients seek from exercise may be unique to them. Although a patient's reasons for being active may differ from the reasons the health care provider considers most important, the patient's reasons, not the health care provider's reasons, drive behavior.

What physical activity do you like or think you would like to do? This question is designed to help guide patients in selecting an appropriate activity that they are motivated to do. A useful strategy is to ask patients to indicate their preference: *1)* long- or short-duration exercise, *2)* high- versus low-intensity exercise, *3)* exercising by themselves or with others, *4)* exercising at home or at a facility, *5)* exercising indoors versus outdoors, or *6)* a competitive or cooperative sport.

Based on the answers to these questions, the health care provider can help identify appropriate activities. Once the patient has chosen a specific activity, the health care provider can encourage consideration of the

"Ease of Access" and "Ease of Performance" indexes. These are self-assessments of how realistic the activity is for a given person.

APPLY THE EASE OF ACCESS AND EASE OF PERFORMANCE INDEXES

Ease of Access Index

A person is more likely to maintain a long-term activity program if it is convenient. Many people begin an exercise program only to find that it is too difficult to maintain for a variety of reasons that were either ignored, rationalized, or simply not considered before beginning the program. To determine patients Ease of Access index for a given activity, ask them to answer the following questions about their chosen activity:

- Does it require special facilities, and are these facilities easily accessible?
- Does it require special equipment, and is this equipment available and affordable?
- Does it require special training, and are training opportunities readily available, scheduled at convenient times, easy to get to, and affordable?
- Does it require others to do it, and will partners always be available?
- Is it seasonal, and are alternate activities available in the off-season?

Ease of Performance Index

To determine how easy it will be for the patient to perform a given activity, ask them the following questions:

Do you have physical limitations that make a given activity unsuitable for you? All people with diabetes should undergo a medical examination to determine whether there are any musculoskeletal or orthopedic concerns that may rule out specific physical activities. Similarly, any existing comorbidities should be identified and considered in the exercise prescription. In addition, a graded exercise test is recommended before beginning an exercise program. The exercise test identifies contraindications to exercise and also facilitates the exercise prescription by establishing safe levels of activity for the individual. To learn more about exercising with diabetes complications, see Table 8.1.

TABLE 8.1 Exercising with Diabetes Complications: Risks and Recommendations

	Retinopathy	Nephropathy	Neuropathy	
			Autonomic	**Peripheral**
Risks	Elevations in blood pressure	Marked changes in hemo-dynamics	Hypoglycemia	Superficial pain
	Possible retina detachment from jarring of head	Marked elevations in blood pressure	Abnormal blood pressure response	Impaired balance/reflexes
		Presence of retinopathy likely	Abnormal heart rate response	Numbness/weakness in hands
			Impaired sympathic/para-sympathic nerves	Decreased proprioception
			Abnormal thermoregulation (prone to dehydration)	Weakness/atrophy of thigh muscles (when severe)
Recommendations	Use heart rate and RPE based on blood pressure response (which should not exceed 170 mmHg systolic; >200 increases damage to retina)	Include dynamic, weight-bearing, low-impact activity	Use submaximal exercise testing	Use RPE to monitor exercise intensity
	Use low-impact activities	Use submaximal isometric or light weight lifting when blood pressure is controlled and left ventricular functioning is normal	Use RPE to gauge exercise intensity	Use non–weight-bearing activities
	Use submaximal exercise testing	Develop specific programs for hemodialysis patients	Use water activities, stationary cycling, or both	Use activities to improve balance
	If possible, monitor blood pressure during exercise			
	Consider stationary cycling, walking, swimming, and low-intensity rowing			

Precautions	Avoid Valsalva maneuvers	Avoid lifting heavy weight,	Avoid high-intensity activity	Examine feet frequently
	Avoid heavy weight lifting,	intense aerobic activities, and	Avoid rapid changes in body	Use proper footwear
	breath-holding stretches,	Valsalva maneuvers	position	Perform gentle, pain-free
	high-intensity exercise,	Use cushioned shoes (gel/air)	Avoid extremes of temperature	stretching
	and strenuous upper arm	Maintain hydration		
	exercise			
	Exercise is contraindicated			
	if recent photo-occulation			
	treatment or surgery has			
	occurred			

Can you realistically integrate regular physical activity into your lifestyle? For many people, the greatest barrier to beginning an exercise program is finding the time to do it. Therefore, when selecting a method of exercise, it is useful to consider "will this fit into my existing schedule or will I have to make special adjustments?"

Can you realistically afford any costs associated with the activity? Many forms of exercise activity require a small, one-time investment. Other activities require a bigger one-time investment, and still others require ongoing fees. Affordable activities are more likely to be maintained over time.

Do you have a good support network? Any activity is easier to engage in if you have the support and encouragement of family and friends. The support needed will vary by person, from active participation, to encouragement, to refraining from being discouraging.

One method to help discuss the Ease of Access and Ease of Performance issues with patients is to have them fill out a brief activity profile. Clinicians can then review patient answers and discuss with them their options. An example of an activity profile is shown in Figure 8.1.

HELP PATIENTS MAINTAIN MOTIVATION

After beginning an exercise program, the challenge is staying with it. Maintaining a program of regular physical activity can be challenging, especially for individuals who have not built a lifelong habit. Moreover, changes in job, family, and other aspects of lifestyle can disrupt the activity program. Therefore, it is important to help people with diabetes maintain their activity program.

The following are a few tips on helping patients maintain their motivation (see Chapter 20 for more information on this subject).

Encourage patients to "play smart." Help your patients understand that the quickest way to destroy their motivation is to injure themselves early in their exercise program. To avoid injuries, patients should stretch properly and warm up before exercising. They should also use proper equipment, especially footwear. Most importantly, patients need to resist the temptation to do too much too fast: a gradual buildup is essential. To "play smart," people need to keep in touch with their diabetes

1. My typical day includes:

   _____ Hours of sleep

   _____ Hours of low activity (driving, reading, watching TV, etc.)

   _____ Hours moderate activity (walking, gardening, housework, etc.)

   _____ Hours vigorous activity (aerobic exercise, heavy labor, competitive sports, etc.)

2. The activities I enjoy most are:

   _____

3. The activities I would like to learn are:

   _____

4. I see the following as obstacles to exercising (check all that apply):

_____ Time	_____ Fear of hypoglycemia	_____ Skills/coordination
_____ Age	_____ Boredom	_____ Energy
_____ Money	_____ Family support	_____ Lack of facilities
_____ Arthritis	_____ Pain during or after exercise	

FIGURE 8.1   Activity profile.

and how their exercise affects it. In particular, individuals who take insulin or medications that increase insulin levels need to understand that increased use of glucose during exercise can result in hypoglycemia during the activity, or even hours later if the activity is intense and lasts a long time. Therefore, it is important that patients know the symptoms of hypoglycemia and always carry some form of quick-acting carbohydrate during exercise sessions.

The health care provider should carefully discuss strategies for adjusting the diabetes regimen for activity, including frequent self-monitoring of blood glucose to learn how different adjustments and types of exercise affect glucose levels. A training log that includes self-monitoring of blood glucose results can help patients remember what did and did not work for them.

Encourage patients to set an activity schedule in advance and stick to it. One of the best ways to keep on track is to set an exercise schedule in advance. Habits are developed through practice. Setting a schedule will help patients avoid scheduling other conflicting activities. Moreover, scheduling helps avoid the "I'll do it later" phenomenon. A regular schedule will also help people to more effectively adjust their regimen so that they will better control their diabetes.

Encourage patients to get a training partner. Many people find that staying active is easier and more enjoyable with a training partner. Partners can be family members, friends, or others committed to improving their health and well-being through activity. If the training partner is not a family member, counsel patients to discuss their diabetes with the partner, including what to do if the patient experiences hypoglycemia.

Encourage patients to set realistic goals. Exercise goals need to be precisely defined and realistically attainable. It is also important that the goals be defined by exercise *behavior* (e.g., walk for 30 min three times per week) rather than defined by an *outcome* of exercise behavior (e.g., lose 20 lb). Encourage patients to set a series of smaller, stepwise goals for which they can observe success and progress (see Chapter 5).

Encourage self-rewards. Progressive rewards for attaining exercise goals help create a more positive reinforcement paradigm that can aid in increasing motivation to stay with the exercise program. Help patients identify rewards to give themselves for accomplishing each goal.

Identify alternative exercise activities to reduce boredom. For some people, having a set routine is the best strategy for exercise adherence. For others, the same activity may eventually become boring, leading to decreased motivation to exercise. Such individuals should "cross-train," i.e., engage in two or more activities that will help them to remain active. The goal, after all, is to do *some* form of exercise.

Accept temporary backslides, but encourage resuming activity. Health care providers should try to understand why patients backslide in their efforts to be more active. Sometimes acknowledging the need for a temporary suspension of activity can be useful if it helps the patient regain the motivation for resuming activity. Encouraging the patient to try a new activity that might be more interesting or less demanding can also be helpful.

Explain the difference between failure and backsliding. Some people set themselves up for failure by ignoring their successes—the "I'm not doing well enough" syndrome. Any deviation from a schedule or failure to meet expectations is viewed as failure. It is important to point out to patients that they should understand and accept that they will have off-days in any long-term exercise program. When they do, it is *not* because they have failed. They are simply having an off-day. Even the most dedicated, world-class athletes have off-days. When your patients do have off-days, remind them they are experiencing a temporary backslide, and help them find ways to get back on track as soon as they can. Encourage patients to tackle the future and not to despair about the past.

Reinforce positive behavior. Any activity is better than none, and for many people with diabetes, even low levels of physical activity are a big accomplishment. Health care professionals are powerful sources of reinforcement for most individuals with diabetes, so always acknowledge efforts to be more active, no matter how limited the efforts may be.

Inquire about physical activity at each visit. The health care provider can reinforce progress and help the patient overcome barriers to maintaining physical activity by inquiring about activity at each visit. This is an opportunity to review the patient's specific motivation for exercise and to adjust the activity program and keep it on track.

Engage family support. Encourage family members to support the patient's activity program. Ideally, activity should become an integral part of family life.

CONCLUSION

Helping patients with diabetes incorporate activity into their daily routine is a significant challenge. This chapter has provided guidelines to help providers meet this challenge. Finally, we recommend that when providers experience periodic frustration with a lack of success in helping patients get more active, they should take a deep breath and relax. Directing this frustration at the patient will not help. Instead, work with the patient to solve the problem. See Chapters 2 and 6 for more on helping patients change behavior and enhancing the provider-patient relationship.

BIBLIOGRAPHY

American College of Sports Medicine. *ACSM's Guidelines for Exercise Testing and Prescription.* 5th ed. Philadelphia, Williams & Wilkins, 1995

American Diabetes Association: Diabetes mellitus and exercise (Position Statement). *Diabetes Care* 22 (Suppl. 1):S49–S53, 1999

American Diabetes Association Council on Exercise: *The Fitness Book for People With Diabetes.* Hornsby WG, Ed. Alexandria, VA, American Diabetes Association, 1994

Campaign B, Lampman RM: *Exercise in the Clinical Management of Diabetes.* Champaign, IL, Human Kinetics, 1994

Herman WH: Leisure-time physical activity patterns in the U.S. diabetic population. *Diabetes Care* 18:27–33, 1995

David G. Marrero, PhD, is Professor of Medicine at Indiana University School of Medicine in Indianapolis, IN. Jill Sizemore, MS, is at the National Insititute for Fitness and Sport in Indianapolis, IN.

9

Improving Weight Loss and Maintenance in Patients with Diabetes

RENA R. WING, PhD

Weight loss is important for patients with diabetes. It is a key component in the management of obese patients with type 2 diabetes, helps in the prevention of diabetes in those with impaired glucose tolerance, and is important in the prevention and/or treatment of weight gain in patients with type 1 diabetes who are using intensive insulin therapy (see Chapter 17).

However, long-term results of most weight control programs are disappointing, and thus, many clinicians have given up even trying to help patients lose weight. This is an example of what psychologists call a self-fulfilling prophecy—if you think you are going to fail, it is very likely you will fail. So, too, if patients embark on weight loss efforts with the expectation that they will be unable to lose weight or to maintain their loss, they are more likely to fail in their efforts.

This chapter provides information and strategies that may help convince clinicians and patients that it is possible to succeed in weight loss. Changing expectations is the first step in changing outcomes.

DECIDE WHO SHOULD LOSE WEIGHT

It is important to determine BMI (weight in kilograms divided by height in meters squared) and waist circumference to identify individuals needing to lose weight.

Weight loss is recommended for all individuals with a BMI >30 and for individuals with a BMI of 25–29.9 or a high-risk waist circumference (>40 inches in men; >35 inches in women) and two or more risk factors. Because type 2 diabetes counts as one risk factor, many individuals with diabetes will be appropriate candidates for weight loss.

SET A REASONABLE GOAL OF LOSING 5–10% OF INITIAL WEIGHT

The average woman entering a weight loss program for individuals with type 2 diabetes weighs 220 lb. Telling this patient that she should achieve her "ideal body weight" is a setup for failure. It is far more reasonable to aim for a weight loss of 5–10% of initial body weight (have the 100-kg woman try to lose 5–10 kg and maintain it).

Such modest weight losses have been shown to produce long-term improvements in glycemic control. In a study of overweight patients with type 2 diabetes, subjects who lost 7–14 kg and maintained it for 1 year had long-term improvement in glycated hemoglobin A1C, insulin, HDL cholesterol, and triglycerides. Likewise, in the Diabetes Prevention Program, a lifestyle intervention that produced weight losses of 5–7 kg reduced the risk of developing diabetes by 58% in individuals with impaired glucose tolerance.

STRESS EXERCISE AS MUCH OR MORE THAN DIET

Exercise is the strongest predictor of long-term maintenance of weight loss. Programs that combine diet plus exercise achieve better long-term weight loss than programs stressing diet or exercise alone. Adding exercise to a diet program also minimizes loss of lean body mass, improves serum lipid profiles, and produces better long-term improvements in glycemic control. Moreover, in studies comparing successful weight losers with those who relapse, the variable that best distinguishes these two groups is the amount of exercise performed.

When recommending exercise to a patient, it is important to set a goal that the patient can achieve (see Chapter 8). We recommend starting slowly, i.e., encouraging the patient to just get out the door for a short walk (10–15 min) on 3 days each week. After the patient achieves this goal for a few weeks, then the distances can be gradually increased until the patient is walking 2 miles per day on 5 days each week. Over time, it may be possible to increase the goal even further.

The goal in weight loss programs is to increase energy expenditure; this goal is best accomplished by increasing the distance walked rather than the speed (or intensity). Walking 1 mile and jogging 1 mile use a similar number of calories. A good rule to remember is the following: **walking 1 mile uses 100 calories.**

Thus, if a patient walks 10 miles each week, he or she will be using an extra 1,000 kcal of energy. Patients can also expend an additional 100 calories by riding a stationary bicycle for 15–30 min, raking leaves for 20 min, weight lifting for 30 min, or playing tennis for 15 min.

It is helpful to encourage patients to set aside a time each day for the purpose of exercise and also to try to increase exercise in their daily routine (such as using stairs instead of elevators). Dividing exercise into multiple short sessions (e.g., four 10-min sessions) may help patients get started. Encourage patients to record their exercise on a daily basis and total it for the week, the month, and the year. These totals help patients see the progress they are making (see Chapter 6).

PRESCRIBE A LOW-FAT/LOW-CALORIE DIET WITH SELF-MONITORING

Several recent studies have suggested that moderate calorie restriction, in combination with a low fat intake, may be the most effective dietary approach for weight loss. When subjects have been taught to limit fat intake only, with no restrictions placed on total calories, weight losses have been modest (2–3 kg). Better results have been achieved when both fat and calories are targeted. Table 9.1 presents an algorithm for determining a calorie and fat goal for patients in a weight loss program.

Self-monitoring of food intake is a key ingredient in teaching patients how to change their dietary intake. In our program, we encourage patients to write down all their food and the calories and grams of fat in each item; these records are kept every day for the first 6 months of treatment and then for at least 1 week each month. Subjects who are most successful at long-term weight control report that they have continued to self-monitor their intake.

Self-monitoring teaches patients a great deal about food. They learn what foods contribute most to their overall calorie and fat intake and how to substitute low-calorie/low-fat foods. Self-monitoring also helps

TABLE 9.1 Setting a Calorie and Fat Goal for a Patient

	Example
1. Estimate patient's current intake by multiplying current weight (in pounds) by 12	200 lb × 12
Estimated current intake =	2,400 calories/day
2. To produce a 1- to 2-lb/week weight loss, prescribe a calorie goal that is 1,000 kcal lower than current intake	2,400 −1,000
Prescribed calorie goal =	1,400 calories/day
3. Determine number of calories from fat for 20% fat intake	1,400 × 0.20
Calories from fat =	280 calories/day
4. Divide calories from fat by 9 to determine number of fat grams to prescribe	280 ÷ 9
Prescribed fat goal =	31 g of fat/day

the patient and provider identify problem areas requiring further attention (e.g., high-calorie desserts, binge-eating episodes).

Another approach to help patients learn to make appropriate food choices is to provide patients with structured menus, indicating exactly what to eat at each meal, and grocery lists, indicating exactly what to purchase. Yet another approach is to provide the actual food that patients should eat, in appropriate portion sizes, during the initial phase of the treatment. Recent studies have shown that such food provision increases weight loss. These strategies also teach subjects more about the number of calories in food and improve the quality of the diet consumed.

CONSIDER VERY-LOW-CALORIE DIETS

Very-low-calorie diets (VLCDs) are diets of <800 kcal/day, usually prescribed as liquid formula or lean meat, fish, and fowl. These diets have been shown to be safe when used with carefully selected patients and appropriate medical monitoring. Such diets can be helpful because they produce fast initial weight losses, averaging 20 kg in 12 weeks, and marked improvements in glycemic control; ~50% of the overall improvement in glycemic control will occur within the first week of starting an 800-kcal diet. These changes can be motivating to patients.

The major disadvantage of VLCDs is that they do not improve the magnitude of weight loss that is maintained long term. Subjects on VLCDs lose more weight initially but then regain more weight than subjects on balanced low-calorie regimens. It remains unclear whether VLCDs promote better long-term glycemic control. If you choose to use VLCDs, keep this in mind, and try to aggressively promote long-term maintenance of weight loss.

KEEP IN CONTACT WITH PATIENTS

Behavioral treatment programs developed in the 1970s usually lasted 10 weeks, and weight losses averaged 4.5 kg. More recently, programs have been increased to 20–24 weeks, and weight losses approximate 9 kg. Some researchers have used longer programs, with weekly meetings for a full year. Although such programs increase overall weight loss, subjects do not maintain a weight loss of 0.5 kg/week, so the cost-effectiveness of lengthening programs beyond 24 weeks becomes increasingly poor. Given this, the current approach is usually to begin treatment with 5–6 months of weekly group treatment.

After 5–6 months of intensive contact, it is important to continue to provide some type of contact for patients. Studies have shown that biweekly meetings involving therapist contact, aerobic exercise, and social support help patients maintain their weight loss. Contact by phone, e-mail, or mail has also been shown to be helpful (see Chapter 5).

IMPLEMENT BEHAVIOR MODIFICATION

It is often said that weight control programs should include diet, exercise, and behavior modification. However, behavior modification is not so much a separate component of a weight loss program as it is a way of understanding and helping patients change their eating and exercise behaviors.

Behavior modification is based on the assumption that behaviors, such as eating and exercise, are learned. Thus, patients can learn new behaviors. Also, it is assumed that behaviors are controlled by the environment, both by *1*) cues in the environment (such as the sight and smell of food) that set the stage for the behavior and by *2*) reinforcers that come after the behavior and lead to its recurrence. Thus, to change behavior, it is important to change the environment that controls it. Key behavioral strategies (see Chapter 7) include self-monitoring to make patients aware of their behaviors, stimulus control techniques and pre-planning to help patients change the environment in which they live, and self-reinforcement and feedback to provide patients with reinforcement for their new behaviors.

CONCLUSION

Weight loss in individuals with diabetes can improve glycemic control and reduce cardiovascular risk factors. The combination of a low-calorie/low-fat diet, physical activity, and behavior modification is most effective for producing and maintaining weight loss.

ACKNOWLEDGMENTS

Preparation of this chapter was supported by National Institutes of Health Grants DK-48412, DK-56992, and HL-41330.

BIBLIOGRAPHY

Diabetes Prevention Program Research Group: Reduction in the incidence of type 2 diabetes with lifestyle intervention or metformin. *N Engl J Med* 346:393–403, 2002

Jeffery RW, Wing RR, Thorson C, Burton LP, Raether C, Harvey J, Mullen M: Strengthening behavioral interventions for weight loss: a randomized trial of food provision and monetary incentives. *J Consult Clin Psychol* 61:1038–1045, 1993

National Institutes of Health/National Heart, Lung, and Blood Institute: *The Practical Guide: Identification, Evaluation, and Treatment of Overweight and Obesity in Adults.* Bethesda, MD, U.S. Department of Health and Human Services, Public Health Service, October 2000 (NIH publ. no. 00-4084)

National Task Force on the Prevention and Treatment of Obesity: Very low-calorie diets. *J Am Med Assoc* 270:967–974, 1993

Perri MG, McAllister DA, Gange JJ, Jordan RC, McAdoo WG, Nezu AM: Effects of four maintenance programs on the long-term management of obesity. *J Consult Clin Psychol* 56:529–534, 1988

Pronk NP, Wing RR: Physical activity and long-term maintenance of weight loss. *Obes Res* 2:587–599, 1994

Wing RR, Koeske R, Epstein LH, Nowalk MP, Gooding W, Becker D: Long-term effects of modest weight loss in type II diabetic patients. *Arch Intern Med* 147:1749–1753, 1987

Rena R. Wing, PhD, is a Professor of Psychiatry and Human Behavior at Brown Medical School/Miriam Hospital in Providence, RI.

10

Smoking Cessation in Diabetes

DEBRA HAIRE-JOSHU, PhD, RN

Cigarette smoking is the greatest source of preventable death in our society, killing over 434,000 people each year, which equals about one of every five deaths. To date, 26–28% of American adults continue to smoke, with variations reported by ethnic and sociodemographic groups. These rates mirror those of individuals with diabetes, who are also less likely to quit smoking than their nondiabetic counterparts. There is evidence of genetic susceptibility to smoking, which, in addition to the biological power of nicotine, makes smokers resistant to change (Table 10.1). Initial studies also suggest that nicotine plays a role in diabetes development and interferes with insulin activity.

Individuals with diabetes who smoke exhibit premature morbidity and mortality; smoking is associated with a heightened incidence of cardiovascular disease and other diabetic complications, including retinopathy, neuropathy, and arterial occlusive disease. For example, among smokers with diabetes, risk for cardiovascular disease is up to 14 times higher than that for smoking or diabetes alone. Nephropathy has been reported as common in patients with type 1 diabetes who smoke, and smoking increases the risk for microalbuminuria in patients with type 2 diabetes. Smoking also increases the risk for neuropathy by 2.2- to 12-fold.

TABLE 10.1 Epidemiology and Special Issues in Smoking and Diabetes

Epidemiology
- The prevalence of smoking among individuals with diabetes is equivalent to that in non-diabetic individuals.
- Only about half of people with diabetes are advised to quit smoking by their health care providers.
- Smoking may increase insulin resistance, interfere with insulin action, and result in poor metabolic control.
- Smoking substantially heightens the risk for neuropathy and nephropathy.
- Smoking significantly enhances the risk for cardiovascular disease, contributing to premature morbidity and mortality.

Special issues
- Postcessation weight gain may be an issue for smokers with diabetes who are focused on weight management. Health care providers should inform the patient of the potential for weight gain but emphasize smoking cessation as the priority for all smokers with diabetes.
- Low mood is associated with increased smoking and decreased cessation rates. Pharmacotherapy for depression should be considered as adjunctive therapy on an as-needed basis for smokers with diabetes.

Adapted from Haire-Joshu D, Glasgow RE, Tibbs TL: Smoking and diabetes (Technical Review). *Diabetes Care* 22:1887–1898, 1999.

The increased risks associated with smoking and diabetes suggest the importance of smoking prevention and cessation as a priority of state-of-the-art diabetes care. Prevention of tobacco use and smoking cessation treatment are cost-effective interventions that should be recommended for all patients with diabetes.

The American Diabetes Association position statement on smoking and diabetes provides clear recommendations for integrating smoking cessation as a primary focus of diabetes management and care. These guidelines are further supported by the recent American Health Care Policy and Research (AHCPR) clinical practice guidelines on treating tobacco use and dependence. The guidelines address three primary areas of practice: assessment, counseling, and effective systems for delivery of smoking cessation.

UNDERSTAND THE GUIDELINE OF ASSESSMENT

Organize the Office Staff and Environment to Emphasize the Importance of Smoking Cessation

Ask about tobacco use at every visit. To effectively do this, it is important to systematically document the history of and current tobacco use for all individuals with diabetes. Table 10.2 reviews steps in completing a smoking cessation assessment. Each setting should have a screening system to ensure that smoking will be consistently assessed and documented in every patient with diabetes (see Chapter 5). A simple system for screening patients' smoking status is to integrate smoking as a vital sign to be checked at each appointment. Posters, clear signage prohibiting smoking, and pamphlets on smoking cessation provide environmental cues that communicate the importance of nonsmoking.

UNDERSTAND THE GUIDELINE OF COUNSELING

Communicate the Importance of Smoking Cessation in Diabetes Care

Health care providers need to encourage smoking prevention and cessation in patients with diabetes. If patients state they do not smoke, **advise** them not to initiate smoking (Table 10.2). This advice is critically important because most adolescents with diabetes who smoke begin using tobacco after they are diagnosed with diabetes. If patients use tobacco, providers need to personalize the message that encourages smoking cessation (see Chapter 15). The reasons for quitting should be made very evident to the patient (e.g., "Quitting smoking is one of the most important things you can do to decrease your risk of developing diabetes complications.").

Communicate an Understanding of the Difficulty of Quitting Smoking

Several failed attempts usually precede successful cessation. Thus, smoking is a chronic problem, like diabetes, that needs to be treated chronically. Promote cessation with recognition that quitting is difficult and with the understanding that the patient's failure to quit is not a sign of lack of concern or interest.

TABLE 10.2 Practice Recommendations Regarding Diabetes and Smoking

Assessment
Ask all patients about their smoking status.
Implement an office-wide system that ensures that for every patient at every clinic visit, tobacco use status is queried and documented. Information should include the answers to the following questions:
- Have you ever smoked?
- Do you smoke now?
- If you previously smoked, when did you quit?

Counseling
Advise all smokers to quit.
In a clear, strong, and personalized manner, urge every tobacco user to quit. Advice should be:
- Clear—"I think it is important for you to quit smoking now, and I can help you. Cutting down while you are ill is not enough."
- Strong—"As your clinician, I need you to know that quitting smoking is the most important thing you can do to protect your health now and in the future. The clinic staff and I will help you."
- Personalized—Tie tobacco use to current health/illness and discuss its social and economic costs, the patient's motivation level/readiness to quit, and/or the impact of tobacco use on children and others in the household.

Ask every tobacco user if he or she is willing to make a quit attempt at this time (e.g., within the next 30 days).

Assess the patient's willingness to quit with the following questions:
- What are your concerns or expectations about quitting?
- Have you thought about quitting? In the next 6 months? In the next month?
- Have you recently quit?

Assist all patients with smoking cessation
If the patient clearly states he or she is unwilling to make a quit attempt at this time, provide a brief motivational intervention encouraging the five "R"s:
- Relevance—Provide individualized information on the hazards of smoking.
- Risks—Emphasize the increased risks of heart disease and diabetes complications that arise from the combination of smoking and diabetes.
- Rewards—Review benefits of smoking cessation: risks of heart disease, especially sudden death, decline within hours of cessation.
- Roadblocks—Assure patients of willingness to assist in their efforts to quit and overcome barriers. Assure patient that prior attempts may encourage future success.
- Repetition—Review patients' thoughts about cessation the next time they come in.

For those thinking about quitting but not ready to quit (i.e., not in the next month):
- Review risks related to diabetes, etc., as above.
- Emphasize that the benefits of quitting clearly outweigh difficulty and costs, especially in terms of heart disease, which is of special importance for people with diabetes.

TABLE 10.2 Continued

- Point out the range of resources for smoking cessation, and help the patient access those resources.
- Express confidence in the patient's ability to quit.

For those about to quit or planning on quitting (e.g., in the next month):
- Review major steps of smoking cessation so that the patient can begin thinking about them.
- Set a quit date appropriate to nature of the habit (i.e., on a weekend if smoking is triggered by work stress).
- Identify likely relapse triggers and make *specific* plans for coping with them *before* quitting.
- Recruit cooperation and encouragement from family and friends.
- Assess and discuss possibility of nicotine replacement.
- Discuss concerns about weight gain and other concerns related to diabetes and how they may be dealt with.
- Encourage the patient to talk with diabetes team or referral resources when ready to make a concrete plan.
- Make referral, prescribe nicotine replacement, provide self-help materials, or otherwise assist in specific plan.

Effective systems for smoking cessation delivery
Arrange for ongoing contact.
- Schedule follow-up contact, either in person or via telephone.
- Follow-up contact should occur soon after the quit date, preferably during the first week.

During follow-up contact, if patient has quit smoking:
- Praise efforts, even if not flawless.
- Encourage vigilance; greatest threat to maintenance may be the myth that, "I'm over the hump, feel pretty good, so I probably can have just a few (at parties, poker games, restaurants, on Wednesday nights, etc.)."
- Review strategies for avoiding triggers; encourage their continuance. It's better to err on the side of caution than recklessness.
- Review plan for support by family/friends or health care team. Provide for team monitoring and encouragement if patient has little other access to these.
- Continue to discuss smoking, and encourage vigilance regarding relapse for at least 6 months, but preferably 1 year.

During follow-up contact, if tobacco use has occurred:
- Congratulate success, review circumstances, and elicit recommitment to total abstinence. Remind patient that a lapse can be used as a learning experience.
- Identify problems already encountered, and anticipate challenges in the immediate future.
- Assess pharmacotherapy use and problems. Consider use or referral to more intensive treatment.

Adapted from Fiore MC, Bailey WC, Cohen SJ, Dorfman SF, Goldstein MG, Gritz ER, et al.: *Treating Tobacco Use and Dependence: Clinical Practice Guideline*. Rockville, MD, U.S. Department of Health and Human Services, Public Health Service, June 2000.

Advise All Patients to Quit Smoking

At each visit, **assess** the willingness of each patient to quit. If patients respond negatively regarding their willingness to quit, motivate them to quit by encouraging the five "R"s: relevance, risks, rewards, roadblocks, and repetition. Remind patients about their personal need to stop smoking in relation to their diabetes and general health. Identify each patient's risk of continued smoking and the immediate benefits of quitting smoking as applied specifically to that patient. Work with the patient to identify any roadblocks to quitting while working on problem-solving solutions to these barriers. At each visit, repeat how important smoking cessation is to the patient's health.

If patients answer affirmatively regarding their willingness to quit, **assist** them by helping develop a plan to quit (described in Table 10.2). In addition, advise patients of the counseling available to them. This counseling includes individual or group sessions and single versus multiple contacts over several weeks. Assess the patient's willingness to engage in minimal counseling (<3 min), brief counseling (3–10 min), or more intensive cessation counseling (including skills training, problem-solving, etc.). Because there is a dose-response relationship between cessation counseling and abstinence, patients should be encouraged to participate in more intensive interventions.

Patients willing to engage in more intensive cessation should be made aware of available smoking cessation community resources. The American Lung Association, the American Heart Association, and the American Cancer Society provide materials for smoking cessation. Local chapters and many hospitals provide group smoking cessation classes and arrange referral procedures.

Consider Pharmacological Supplements for Promoting Smoking Cessation

All smokers with diabetes should be offered pharmacological supplements for use as an adjunct to behavioral counseling interventions, except in special circumstances such as pregnancy. Pharmacological supplements are effective when combined with behavioral counseling interventions for smoking cessation. Nicotine replacement and other pharmacological therapies allow patients to split quitting into two tasks: *1*) getting accustomed to life without all the smoking habits they have developed and *2*) giving up nicotine altogether. According to the recent AHCPR guidelines, five first-line pharmacotherapies have been identified as reliably increasing long-term smoking abstinence. These first-line pharmacotherapy medications include bupropion SR (sustained release), nicotine gum, nicotine inhaler, nicotine nasal spray, and nicotine patch.

Encourage Cessation Maintenance

Cessation symptoms include acute cravings, irritability, lethargy (or increased energy), difficulty concentrating, headache, and changes in blood glucose. Reassure patients that these symptoms will pass within 3–10 days, and provide practical tips for avoiding them. Encourage patients to use their own common sense in combating withdrawal symptoms while reassuring them that such symptoms are normal and not a sign of impending failure.

Frequent causes of initial relapse include environmental triggers (social situations, habitual smoking cues, pressure from peers), psychological triggers (negative moods, stress, low motivation to remain abstinent), and physiological cravings or withdrawal symptoms. Self-management strategies may minimize relapse triggers and vary according to the situation. For example, identify that the trigger is telephone conversations with friends, not just being on the phone. Suggest strategies to avoid triggers before the triggers gain control (e.g., go for a walk rather than sit at the far end of the table away from smokers during a coffee break). Finally, work with the patient to identify strategies to restrict choices to smoke (e.g., go to a restaurant that doesn't allow smoking, so that after-dinner coffee and a cigarette won't be such a temptation).

Address Weight Gain

Emphasis on weight maintenance may cause those with diabetes to fear weight gain after smoking cessation. Assure the patient that the risk of smoking far outweighs the risk of the average 5- to 10-lb weight gain, even for those with diabetes. When encouraging smoking cessation, be sure to acknowledge that few patients will be able to quit smoking at the same time as focusing on weight management (see Chapter 9). It may be helpful to acknowledge that previous emphasis on weight in diabetes care may have drawn attention away from the importance of smoking cessation. Reassure patients that once nonsmoking status is secure, they can work out a plan for losing the gained weight. Encourage the patient to continue to exercise because activity limits weight gain, promotes diabetes management, and can distract the quitter from urges to smoke.

It is not clear when to return to a focus on weight management. The rate of relapse to smoking is especially high through most of the first 6 months after quitting but levels off between 6 and 12 months. A helpful guideline is that patients should not limit eating until they can do so without any noticeable desire to smoke. Otherwise, patients may be on a merry-go-round of quitting smoking, gaining weight, returning to smoking to lose the weight, quitting smoking, gaining weight, and so on.

Address Emotional Factors Related to Smoking and Diabetes

Smoking reduces anxiety and elevates mood and can be especially useful for individuals dealing with the stressors of diabetes. Additionally, smokers with diabetes report reluctance to give up the pleasures of smoking amidst all the other pleasures they see themselves as giving up because of their diabetes. Health care providers should address the influence of these effects on a patient's ability to quit and maintain abstinence from smoking. If the patient has been treated for mood disturbance or depression, the professional providing that care might be consulted. Or, if the patient relies heavily on smoking to manage mood, referral for counseling may be helpful. If possible, have this counseling provided by someone with experience in smoking cessation.

Discuss the Risk of Relapse

Long-term quitters frequently say that the most important thing they learned from their earlier failures was that they could not have "just one" and that, in the long run, it is easier simply to abstain than to try to control the addiction. Those who slip or relapse in the first weeks after quitting are far less likely to remain abstinent. It is important to encourage a clear determination not even to have "just one." On the other hand, it is also important to reinforce the patient's efforts if a lapse does occur and to encourage resumption of the quit attempt. Many who have had relapses have gone on to success (see Chapter 7).

Remind patients that most long-term quitters have failed two to three times before succeeding. Encourage patients who have lapsed to review the details of the lapse situation and identify specific things they want to do differently the next time.

UNDERSTAND THE GUIDELINE OF EFFECTIVE SYSTEMS FOR DELIVERY OF SMOKING CESSATION

Arrange for Ongoing Contact

Ongoing follow-up and patient support are critical to long-term smoking abstinence (Table 10.2). Follow up with a visit or phone call several days after the quit date, and then make several more contacts during the first several weeks. Thereafter, decrease contacts from biweekly to monthly to bimonthly, but continue contacts for at least 6 months. Because repetition of contact is important, staff can develop procedures for this that suit the practice setting and their own strengths.

Contribute to the Overall Campaign to Promote Nonsmoking

Smoking cessation is accomplished not through any single strategy but through a combination of multiple strategies. First, providers should assist with public health, community, and mass media campaigns that encourage smoking cessation. For instance, an American Diabetes Association affiliate might cosponsor a program on smoking cessation on a local television news channel and encourage individuals with diabetes to organize their own quit efforts around the television program. Or, an affiliate might promote locally available smoking cessation resources to its members.

Second, all health care providers should be aware of, and trained, to implement the guidelines for smoking cessation identified by the AHCPR. This training ensures consistency in methods that have been shown effective in preventing smoking and promoting cessation and long-term abstinence.

ACKNOWLEDGMENTS

Edwin B. Fisher Jr., PhD, and Sheryl L. Ziff, MA, were coauthors for this chapter in the first edition of *Practical Psychology for Diabetes Clinicians*.

BIBLIOGRAPHY

Ahluwalia JS, Gibson CA, Kenney RE, Wallace DD, Resnicow K: Smoking status as a vital sign. *J Gen Intern Med* 14:402–408, 1999

American Diabetes Association: Smoking and diabetes (Position Statement). *Diabetes Care* 23 (Suppl. 1):S63–S64, 2000

Fiore MC, Bailey WC, Cohen SJ, Dorfman SF, Goldstein MG, Gritz ER, et al.: *Treating Tobacco Use and Dependence: Clinical Practice Guideline.* Rockville, MD, U.S. Department of Health and Human Services, Public Health Service, June 2000

Haire-Joshu D, Glasgow RE, Tibbs TL: Smoking and diabetes (Technical Review). *Diabetes Care* 22:1887–1898, 1999

Haire-Joshu D, Glasgow RE, Tibbs TL: Smoking and diabetes. *Pract Diabetol* 20:16–28, 2001

Debra Haire-Joshu, PhD, RN, is a Professor of Behavioral Science and Director of the Obesity Prevention Center at Saint Louis University School of Public Health in St. Louis, MO.

11

Helping Patients Understand, Recognize, and Avoid Hypoglycemia

LINDA A.GONDER-FREDERICK, PhD,
DANIEL J. COX, PhD,
AND WILLIAM L. CLARKE, MD

Hypoglycemia occurs when glucose levels in the bloodstream drop too low to maintain normal body and brain function. In type 1 diabetes, low blood glucose (BG) (<70 mg/dl) is caused by an excess of insulin relative to food intake and/or physical activity. Because hypoglycemia can be so frightening and potentially dangerous to patients, it is considered one of the major barriers to obtaining and maintaining good diabetes control.

Hypoglycemic episodes can be classified as mild or severe (Table 11.1). These classifications are not based an any particular BG level but rather on whether *1)* severe neuroglycopenia occurs and *2)* the patient is able to self-treat. Neuroglycopenia occurs when glucose levels in the brain drop too low to maintain normal function.

It is impossible to say that severe hypoglycemia occurs at any specific BG level because of the individual differences in the glycemic threshold for physiological reactions and symptoms. Whereas some patients become very symptomatic at BG levels of 60 mg/dl, others show few symptoms at BG levels <50 mg/dl. It is important for individual patients to know their personal threshold for hypoglycemic symptoms.

It is also important to emphasize that the term "mild" does not mean that a hypoglycemic episode is inconsequential or that patients only experience mild symptoms. It simply means that the patient did not

TABLE 11.1 Hypoglycemic Episodes

Mild
- Symptoms can include shaking, sweating, and slowed thinking
- Patient can self-treat
- Symptoms disappear with self-treatment

Severe
- Severe neuroglycopenic symptoms (lethargy, mental stupor, unconsciousness)
- Patient unable to self-treat because of neuroglycopenia

become *so severely* neuroglycopenic that he or she was unable to self-treat. From the patient's perspective, even mild hypoglycemia can be quite aversive and cause unpleasant symptoms, disruptions in planned activities, and social embarrassment (see Chapter 1).

Almost all patients taking insulin experience mild hypoglycemic episodes periodically. Although hypoglycemia is typically more problematic in patients with type 1 diabetes who are insulin dependent, it also occurs in patients with type 2 diabetes who are taking insulin or medications that raise insulin levels. Whereas much research has focused on hypoglycemia in patients with type 1 diabetes, much less is known about hypoglycemia in patients with type 2 diabetes. However, a recent study of a large sample of patients with type 2 diabetes found that 3.2% of BG readings were <70 mg/dl and 1% were <54 mg/dl. In both type 1 and type 2 diabetes, hypoglycemia is especially problematic when using intensive insulin regimens (i.e., multiple daily injections or an insulin pump).

Severe hypoglycemic episodes are less common. However, there are many patients who have frequent and recurrent episodes, and even one episode can be traumatic and potentially dangerous. If severe hypoglycemia occurs, for example, when patients are performing critical tasks—such as driving a car, caring for children, or operating dangerous equipment—serious injury, and even death, can occur.

UNDERSTAND WHY PATIENTS FEAR HYPOGLYCEMIA

It is not surprising that many patients have considerable fear and anxiety about the possibility of hypoglycemia and its negative consequences.

Sometimes this fear can result in inappropriate treatment, such as behaviors that keep BG in a higher, "safer" range. Table 11.2 lists patients who are at high risk for developing fear of hypoglycemia.

Family members and friends can also develop fear of hypoglycemia. Parents who have a young child with diabetes often show high levels of fear, especially when the child has experienced unconsciousness due to hypoglycemia (see Chapter 12). Spouses and partners of adult patients who have recurrent severe hypoglycemia also show high levels of fear. In both children and adults, fear of hypoglycemia can create tension and conflict in relationships. For example, after a traumatic episode, spouses or parents can become overprotective and hypervigilant, which can be resented by the patient.

Some patients have a strong fear of hyperglycemia because they are extremely worried about long-term complications. This fear can lead to overtreating high BG levels by taking more insulin than is necessary, which can cause hypoglycemia.

UNDERSTAND HYPOGLYCEMIC SYMPTOMS

There are two primary methods for detecting hypoglycemia: *1*) self-testing of BG and *2*) feeling physical symptoms. Because most patients typically measure their BG only a few times each day, the majority of hypoglycemic episodes occur when patients are not testing. The onset of hypoglycemia can occur quite suddenly. For this reason, patients strongly rely on symptoms to tell them when their BG is too low. Patients' ability to self-treat in a timely manner and avoid severe hypo-

TABLE 11.2

Patients at High Risk for Fear of Hypoglycemia

- Newly diagnosed patients who have not yet learned that they can deal with hypoglycemia
- Patients who have had a recent or past traumatic episode
- Patients who tend to be overly anxious in other areas of their lives
- Patients who live alone
- Patients whose job/career could be negatively affected by hypoglycemia (e.g., truck drivers, airline pilots)

glycemia depends greatly on their ability to recognize early warning symptoms accurately.

Most hypoglycemic symptoms fall into one of two categories—autonomic or neuroglycopenic. Autonomic symptoms are caused by hormonal counterregulation, primarily epinephrine secretion, which raises BG by stimulating the liver to release stored glucose. These symptoms include trembling, sweating, and heart palpitations.

This epinephrine response can be reduced by many different factors, including caffeine and alcohol consumption, frequency of low BG episodes, metabolic control, and autonomic neuropathy. For this reason, the degree to which adequate counterregulation occurs differs across both individual patients and different episodes of hypoglycemia. Patients who experience frequent and extreme low BG levels, for example, have a weaker and delayed counterregulatory response. This has the unfortunate effect of reducing the intensity of autonomic symptoms and/or delaying their onset, which, in turn, greatly increases the risk of severe hypoglycemia.

Patients are typically not well educated about neuroglycopenic symptoms and are not taught to use them as early warning cues. Traditionally, neuroglycopenia was believed to occur only with severe hypoglycemia, but we now know that it can occur when BG is only mildly low (<65 mg/dl). Patients often recognize the subtle impairments in mental and motor abilities that occur with early neuroglycopenia. These include difficulty concentrating, slowed thinking, lightheadedness or dizziness, and lack of coordination.

The degree to which individual patients experience neuroglycopenia varies greatly. Some patients become quite symptomatic with mild hypoglycemia, whereas others show few signs of impairment, even with very low BG. Patients who experience frequent hypoglycemia tend to become more neuroglycopenic than those who do not and may also have more difficulty in recognizing their impairment—a potentially dangerous combination.

Patients who are extremely vulnerable to neuroglycopenia should avoid BG levels <70 mg/dl. This may require changes in the treatment regimen, such as eating or drinking carbohydrates when BG levels are <80 mg/dl.

Both epinephrine secretion and neuroglycopenia can cause a variety of different physiological responses and symptoms. Table 11.3 lists some of the most common.

TABLE 11.3

Symptoms of Hypoglycemia

Autonomic symptoms	Neuroglycopenic symptoms	Mood changes
• Trembling/shaking	• Slowed thinking	• Nervous/tense
• Pounding heart	• Lightheadedness/dizziness	• Jittery
• Fast pulse	• Trouble concentrating	• Irritated
• Flushed face	• Slurred speech	• Worried
• Sweating	• Blurred vision	• Frustrated
• Temperature changes	• Difficulty reading or talking	• Angry
• Queasy stomach	• Sleepiness	• Distressed
• Weakness	• Numbness	• Sad/unhappy
• Tingling	• Lack of coordination	• Stubborn
• Headache		• Giddy
• Heavy/rapid breathing		• Euphoric

UNDERSTAND THE RELATIONSHIP BETWEEN HYPOGLYCEMIA AND MOOD CHANGES

As Table 11.3 shows, in addition to physical symptoms and disruptions in mental/motor abilities, many patients experience mood changes with hypoglycemia. These mood changes can range from feelings of mild anxiety and irritability to outright anger and belligerence, and even to feelings of giddiness. Individual patients differ greatly in their tendency to experience emotions with hypoglycemia. Both hormonal counterregulation and neuroglycopenia contribute to these mood changes.

Hypoglycemia tends to intensify moods that are already occurring. For this reason, patients need to monitor themselves for mood changes and emotional responses that seem out of proportion to whatever event is occurring.

Sometimes, positive moods occur with hypoglycemia, but usually the emotional changes are negative. The negative mood changes caused by hypoglycemia can create interpersonal tension, embarrassment, and even conflict. One patient, for example, reported that she was often embarrassed by the "evil twin who appears" when she is hypoglycemic. These mood changes can also interfere with others' ability to assist during hypoglycemia, when patients become resistant and refuse treatment.

The stress that hypoglycemia-related mood changes can place on relationships is often clinically neglected. To help patients identify these problems, ask a few direct, but nonjudgmental, questions (e.g., "Does hypoglycemia ever affect your emotions or your moods?" or "Has this ever caused you to have problems in relationships, like arguments, with others?") (see Chapter 19).

HELP PATIENTS RECOGNIZE HYPOGLYCEMIC SYMPTOMS

All patients do not experience the same symptoms, and, in fact, hypoglycemic symptoms tend to be quite idiosyncratic. This means that the most reliable symptoms for one patient will not be the most reliable for another patient. For this reason, it is critical for patients to identify their own best *personal* warning symptoms.

Patients do not, however, always recognize and interpret hypoglycemic symptoms accurately. There are three psychological barriers to accurate symptom perception:

1. Inattentiveness
2. Inaccurate symptom beliefs
3. Misattribution of symptoms

Inattentiveness occurs when patients are distracted, attending to a competing demand, or intensely focused on a task. Patients can also actively avoid paying attention to symptoms because they do not want to interrupt an enjoyable or productive activity.

Some patients have inaccurate or "false alarm" symptom beliefs. These are symptoms that patients believe are reliable signs of hypoglycemia but are, in reality, often independent of BG. Symptoms that tend to be false alarms are hunger and fatigue, which are just as likely to occur with normal or high BG. Patients high in trait anxiety (predisposition to experience anxiety in numerous areas of life) often believe their anxiety-related symptoms are due to low BG when they are not.

Sometimes patients misattribute symptoms that are related to hypoglycemia to some other cause. For example, a patient exercising may think that his or her sweating is due to exertion rather than hypoglycemia.

HELP PATIENTS TO IMPROVE THEIR ABILITY TO RECOGNIZE HYPOGLYCEMIC SYMPTOMS

Patients can be taught to recognize the symptoms of hypoglycemia more accurately and to reduce the frequency of episodes. Over the past

20 years, our research team has developed the intervention of blood glucose awareness training (BGAT), which improves the ability to detect and avoid both hypoglycemia and hyperglycemia. Some of the techniques used in BGAT can be applied in any clinical setting. (Information on how to purchase the BGAT training manual can be obtained from the first author at the Behavioral Medicine Center, Box 800223, University of Virginia Health System, Charlottesville, VA 22908; e-mail: lag3g@virginia.edu. An interactive BGAT web site that will allow patients to undergo BGAT at home is in development.)

For example, the BGAT diary (Figure 11.1) can help clinicians obtain an *objective* assessment of the patient's ability to detect hypoglycemia and of which symptoms most reliably co-occur with low BG levels. To use the diary, patients simply *1*) "scan" themselves for any symptoms and record these, *2*) record recent insulin, food, or physical activity if the patient believes these could be causing low BG, *3*) estimate current BG level based on all of these "cues," and *4*) measure and record actual BG level.

After doing this for 1 week or more (at least 50 entries), the diary can be reviewed. If hypoglycemic awareness is being assessed, however, the patient must keep the diary long enough to have at least four to five actual BG readings <70 mg/dl to have enough information about ability to detect low BG levels. The number of times the patient detected low BG should be counted to assess his or her ability to recognize hypoglycemia (count both actual and estimated BG <70 mg/dl). For example, patients with very poor hypoglycemic awareness will have few, if any, estimated BG readings <70 mg/dl, even when actual BG readings are quite low. Then count the number of times each symptom occurred when BG levels were <70 and >120 mg/dl, i.e., count the times the symptom occurred with low BG and with normal to high BG. For example, it is often found that symptoms such as "hunger" or "tired" occur just as often when BG is in a normal or even high range as they do when BG is low. Thus, the diary gives a measure of how *sensitive* and *specific* a symptom is to hypoglycemia. The best symptoms are those that are both sensitive and specific, i.e., they occur mostly when BG is low and rarely when it is not. If analysis of the diary yields inconclusive information, the patient can continue making diary entries for another 2 weeks or longer to obtain more data on specific BG levels and symptoms.

We also recommend that clinicians teach patients to use neuroglycopenic symptoms as early warning signs of hypoglycemia. To do this,

Cues: Scan your body for dryness in mouth and nose or changes in your: thinking, vision, taste, balance, sweating, breathing, heart rate, coordination, urination, hunger, energy, tension, tolerance, insulin, food, activity, others.

BGAT Diary Sheet

Name: _____

Date	Time	I	F	E	Symptoms and Performance Cues	Estimate	Actual	Missed	Opportunities/Treatment

First, list the date and time of each entry. I, F, and E refer to your most recent insulin, food, and exercise. In each of these columns, write M, L, or U if you took more, less, or your usual amount of insulin, food, and exercise. Next, write in any BG cues you might have, including any symptoms, disruptions in routine performance, time of day, whether you recently had low BG, whether your insulin is peaking, etc. Based on these BG cues, estimate your BG and write that in the Estimate column. Next, measure and record your actual BG in the Actual column. If your BG was low (<70 mg/dl) and you did not recognize this, ask yourself, "What cues did I miss and why?" Write down the cues you missed in the Missed column and why you missed them in the Opportunities/Treatment column.

After 30–50 entries, take a yellow marker and highlight all those times when your actual BG was <70 mg/dl. When your BG was low, were you more likely to take more insulin, eat less, or exercise more compared with when you were not low? What symptoms occurred only when you were low? What percent of the time did you recognize when you were low? When you failed to recognize low BG, what cues did you miss that you can look for in the future?

FIGURE 11.1 BGAT Diary Sheet

encourage patients to monitor their ability to think clearly and perform routine tasks. When BG is low, patients may notice that they are thinking or moving more slowly and that they have to exert more effort to do simple tasks such as reading, following conversations, or typing. Table 11.4 lists questions patients can use to help recognize these symptoms.

Almost all hypoglycemia is caused by treatment decisions and behaviors, and it is critical to help patients improve their ability to predict and avoid episodes. In BGAT, patients compare their insulin action curves with their food and physical activity to identify times of day and specific situations when they are likely to become low. Patients may not fully understand how changing the timing or dose of insulin affects food requirements or that *any* significant increase in physical activity (not just "exercise") can lower BG.

Encourage patients to monitor symptoms carefully, especially at times when their BG is more likely to be low (when insulin is peaking, less food has been eaten, or physical activity has increased). Teaching patients to respond appropriately and immediately to hypoglycemia is equally important. Many episodes of severe hypoglycemia are caused by delaying treatment or by using high-fat foods, such as candy bars, which increase BG slowly compared with high-carbohydrate, low-fat foods.

LEARN ABOUT HYPOGLYCEMIC UNAWARENESS

Patients with dampened or delayed autonomic symptoms, called hypoglycemic unawareness, are at much higher risk for severe hypoglycemia and require special clinical attention. There is now strong evidence that hypoglycemic unawareness is sometimes reversible. Autonomic symptoms increase when patients meticulously avoid low BG (<70 mg/dl).

TABLE 11.4 Questions Patients Can Use to Check Themselves for Neuroglycopenia

Compared with my usual ability:
- Am I performing this task more slowly?
- Is it taking more effort to perform this task?
- Does this task seem more difficult than usual?
- Am I making more mistakes?
- In general, how impaired do I feel?

However, because this strategy can jeopardize metabolic control, patients must be closely followed.

We also recommend that clinicians rule out the possibility that these patients have symptoms that they are not aware of. Patients who are classified as hypoglycemic unaware rarely have *no* symptoms: they have *reduced* symptoms. Our research shows that patients presumed to be hypoglycemic unaware improve their ability to detect hypoglycemia when they undergo BGAT.

When patients report reduced awareness of hypoglycemia, use the BGAT diary. This procedure will help to identify reliable symptoms and often increases patient attentiveness to symptoms as well. Teach and encourage these patients to use mild neuroglycopenic symptoms as early warning signs of hypoglycemia.

LEARN TO TALK TO PATIENTS ABOUT HYPOGLYCEMIA

Some patients are reluctant to talk to clinicians about hypoglycemia. They may fear being blamed for "doing something wrong" or other negative consequences, such as losing their license to drive, or be embarrassed by their behavior during episodes. Thus, clinicians may not even be aware when hypoglycemia is a significant problem.

Patients are especially reluctant to talk about hypoglycemia and driving problems, and clinicians often fail to inquire about this important topic. Impaired driving can occur with BG levels <65 mg/dl, and many patients mistakenly believe that it is safe to drive with mild hypoglycemia. Patients need to be *1*) warned about the danger of driving when BG is low, *2*) encouraged to self-test before driving, *3*) instructed to pull off the road immediately and self-treat if hypoglycemia occurs while driving, and *4*) advised not to resume driving until BG and mental/motor abilities return to normal.

To increase dialogue with patients about hypoglycemia, it is helpful to adopt a nonjudgmental, collaborative, and problem-solving approach (see Chapters 1 and 2). Table 11.5 discusses ways to help clinicians better assess hypoglycemia-related issues and the need for intervention.

CONCLUSION

Hypoglycemia is a major problem for many patients with diabetes. In addition to placing patients at physical risk, hypoglycemia can have seri-

TABLE 11.5 How to Facilitate Discussions About Hypoglycemia-Related Problems

Ask patients about:
- Frequency of episodes, especially severe hypoglycemia
- Possible causes of episodes (look for self-treatment behaviors that contributed, e.g., delaying treatment, skipping meals)
- Frequency of increased insulin doses at meals without considering carbohydrate intake
- Negative consequences (injury, embarrassment, interpersonal conflict)
- Worry/fear about future hypoglycemia
- Any changes in self-treatment or actions they currently take to avoid hypoglycemia (look for behaviors that keep BG higher)
- Personal symptom cues, thresholds, and beliefs
- Ability to recognize hypoglycemia
- Frequency of asymptomatic hypoglycemia, any symptoms that have disappeared or occur at a lower threshold
- Vulnerability to neuroglycopenic symptoms and mental stupor
- Habits/beliefs concerning driving ability and hypoglycemia

ous psychosocial consequences. These include extreme fear of hypoglycemia and conflicts in relationships (see Chapter 23). Patients rely on symptoms to warn them when BG is too low. Because both the type and intensity of hypoglycemic symptoms vary from patient to patient, it is important to help each patient identify his or her own best *personal* warning cues. In addition to the classic autonomic symptoms (trembling, sweating), patients need to be taught to monitor neuroglycopenic symptoms and mood changes as signs of low BG. Clinicians can objectively assess patients' symptoms and ability to detect hypoglycemia by using a BG diary in which patients record their symptoms, estimated BG levels, and BG self-tests results. Patients who may especially benefit from this type of assessment include those who report reduced hypoglycemic symptoms and those who have problems with recurrent severe hypoglycemia. Clinicians can also help patients better cope with hypoglycemia by assessing problem areas and maintaining an open dialogue about this important topic, including discussions concerning driving and low BG.

ACKNOWLEDGMENTS

This work was supported in part by grants from the National Institutes of Health (R01-DK-28288 and RR-00847).

BIBLIOGRAPHY

Clarke WL, Cox DJ, Gonder-Frederick LA, Kovatchev BP: Hypoglycemia and the decision to drive a motor vehicle by persons with diabetes. *JAMA* 282:750–754, 1999

Cox DJ, Gonder-Frederick LA, Kovatchev BP, Julian DM, Clarke WL: Progressive hypoglycemia's impact on driving simulation performance: occurrence, awareness and correction. *Diabetes Care* 23:163–170, 2000

Cox DJ, Gonder-Frederick LA, Polonsky WH, Schlundt DG, Kovatchev BP, Clarke WL: Blood glucose awareness training (BGAT-2): long-term benefits. *Diabetes Care* 24:637–642, 2001

Gonder-Frederick LA, Clarke WL, Cox DJ: The emotional, social, and behavioral implications of insulin-induced hypoglycemia. *Semin Clin Neuropsychiatry* 2:57–65, 1997

Gonder-Frederick LA, Cox DJ, Kovatchev BP, Schlundt D, Clarke WL: A biopsychobehavioral model of risk of severe hypoglycemia. *Diabetes Care* 20:661–669, 1997

Kovatchev BP, Cox DJ, Gonder-Frederick LA, Clarke WL: Methods for quantifying self-monitoring blood glucose profiles exemplified by an examination of blood glucose patterns in patients with type 1 and type 2 diabetes. *Diabetes Technologies and Therapeutics.* In press

---

Linda A. Gonder-Frederick, PhD, is an Associate Professor, Daniel J. Cox, PhD, is a Professor, and William L. Clarke, MD is a Professor, all in the Department of Pediatric Medicine at the University of Virginia Health System in Charlottesville, VA.

Three

Responding to Developmental and Family Influences on Self-Care

Developmental and family factors dramatically affect diabetes care, just as they affect the risk of developing diabetes in the first place. Chapters in this part are designed to help clinicians work more effectively with family issues in diabetes care and with patients in some of the more challenging age-groups: children, adolescents, young adults, and the elderly. We also include chapters on preventing type 2 diabetes in both children and adults.

In the first chapter, Delamater provides practical recommendations for the care of children who have diabetes. The author describes how to work with young children and their parents to develop a plan for family management of diabetes.

Next, Rubin presents guidelines for working with adolescents; these guidelines focus on helping teenagers to deal with their feelings and to make more healthy self-care choices in diabetes management. Rubin offers strategies for maintaining partnerships between adolescents and clinicians as well as partnerships between adolescents and their parents.

Wolfsdorf discusses the key factors involved in improving glycemic control during adolescence. These efforts are fueled by the documented benefits of closer-to-normal blood glucose levels. The author offers suggestions for facilitating improved glycemic control in teenagers who have diabetes.

Young adulthood—a time when many older adolescents transition away from home to start jobs or to continue their education or training—is a critical period for diabetes management. The combination of competing priorities and separation from familiar sources of health care and support can compromise diabetes care and outcomes. In his chapter, Wolpert describes the challenges and opportunities of working with young adults who have diabetes. He also offers practical guidelines for helping young adults make wise decisions about diabetes care.

Recent years have seen an alarming increase in the number of children and adolescents diagnosed with type 2 diabetes. This condition, relatively unknown 20 years ago, now accounts for a substantial proportion of all youth diagnosed with diabetes. Many young people who develop type 2 diabetes are members of racial/ethnic minorities. In her chapter, Young-Hyman provides recommendations for identifying youth at risk for type 2 diabetes, along with suggestions for interventions to reduce this risk. These recommendations reflect the need to address social, cultural, and economic issues in patients' lives.

The epidemic of type 2 diabetes among people of all ages appears to be fueled largely by widespread changes in lifestyle: in many countries all over the world, people are eating more, especially more saturated fats, and they are less active. In her chapter, Walker discusses the promising results of diabetes prevention efforts, including the recently concluded Diabetes Prevention Program. The author offers practical guidelines for clinicians who want to help their patients reduce the risk of developing type 2 diabetes.

Zrebiec discusses the many complicated and interrelated physical and psychological challenges facing elderly patients with diabetes. He provides suggestions for giving optimal and sensitive care to these patients.

In the last chapter of this part, B. Anderson offers practical guidelines for working with families of patients with diabetes—whether the patient is a child, a young adult, or an older adult. Specific recommendations allow the clinician to help families learn how to be truly helpful to their loved ones who have diabetes.

12

Working with Children Who Have Type 1 Diabetes

ALAN M. DELAMATER, PhD, ABPP

Successful management of diabetes is always challenging, especially when working with children. Epidemiological studies indicate that the incidence of type 1 diabetes has increased in recent years, particularly among young children. This chapter presents treatment guidelines and principles of intervention.

UNDERSTAND THE TREATMENT GUIDELINES

Help Children and Parents Manage Critical Issues at Diagnosis

The diagnosis of type 1 diabetes represents a crisis for both children and parents. Both must:

- accept the diagnosis and its implications in a realistic way
- manage their own psychological response to the diagnosis
- learn a new set of complex skills relating to diabetes management
- not allow diabetes to interfere with the attainment of normal developmental tasks

Studies have shown that in the initial period of adaptation after diagnosis, a significant number of children and parents (particularly mothers) become depressed and anxious. In most cases, these reactions subside within the first year. However, if adjustment problems persist, there is a greater risk for later problems with psychosocial adjustment and glycemic control (see Chapter 20). Besides having to acquire a lot of new knowledge about diabetes and its management, parents and children must master new skills and figure out how to integrate diabetes management into daily life.

Help Parents Have Realistic Expectations Concerning Their Children's Responsibility for Self-Management

Parents of very young children assume all responsibilities for diabetes management. Over time, however, children can begin to assume some responsibilities for certain aspects of self-care. Learning to identify who is responsible for what tasks at what times is an important issue for families because studies have shown that disagreements about these responsibilities are related to poor glycemic control.

Some research has found that parents and clinicians disagree in their estimates of the age at which children are ready for self-care independence. Findings indicate that certain self-management behaviors (insulin adjustment, in particular) depend on cognitive maturity rather than age. Glycemic control problems are more likely when children are given self-care responsibilities that they are not yet able to handle competently.

Help Parents Facilitate Good Self-Care Attitudes and Behaviors in Their Children

Several studies of older children and adolescents have demonstrated that poor communication skills and family conflict are associated with problems of regimen adherence and glycemic control. Parents and their children must strive for effective communication to avoid and resolve conflicts. In addition, parents and children must develop a good relationship with their health care team. A good relationship, based on trust and support, will foster agreement and understanding about exactly what the parents and children are supposed to do to manage diabetes effectively. It is critical that families and health care providers agree on what the goals of diabetes management are and what specific regimens are prescribed. It is very important that children and their parents have regular meetings with the health care team because studies have shown that children who have more regular and frequent appointments attain better metabolic control than those who do not. Maintaining contact with the health care team between clinic visits, via telephone and/or e-mail, may also help to facilitate effective diabetes management. Health care providers should also be alert to the special needs of minority families and children from lower income groups who live in single-parent families because research has shown that these children are at increased risk for poor metabolic control (see Chapter 4).

Help Parents and Children Learn to Avoid and Treat Hypoglycemia

Studies have shown that children who are diagnosed before 5 years of age and who have more episodes of serious hypoglycemia may be at increased risk for later neurocognitive problems. Such children should receive psycho-educational evaluations for early identification of learning problems. Because of this potential complication and the fact that young children cannot verbalize their subjective experience of hypoglycemia, parents may feel highly stressed about hypoglycemia. Thus, parents need to monitor their child's blood glucose frequently to assure themselves that their child is not hypoglycemic. Common psychological reactions of parents and children to frequent blood glucose monitoring may include feelings of anger for the child, guilt for the parent, and distress for both.

Help Parents and Children Develop Realistic Attitudes Toward Glycemic Control

Parents may get in the habit of giving evaluative messages to their children regarding the results of blood glucose monitoring. Hyperglycemia and hypoglycemia may be seen as "bad" readings. When viewed in this way, such readings are less likely to be used as feedback to solve problems and try new strategies.

Help patients use the information they collect on a daily basis to gain a better understanding of blood glucose variations; to make appropriate changes in insulin dose, diet, and activity; and to solve problems related to glycemic control.

Parents and children may be anxious about insulin injections and dose adjustments. After an injection, many children may not want to eat within an appropriate time, causing parents to be concerned about hypoglycemia, particularly when using a new fast-acting insulin. Many young children are finicky eaters, making meal planning very challenging. Counsel parents to tell children ahead of time when meals will be served. This can be done while administering insulin. Encourage parents to then reinforce their children for eating at the appropriate time. When children do not consume their food within the appropriate time, consideration may be given to administering a fast-acting insulin when the meal is complete.

New research indicates that the insulin dose should optimally match the amount of carbohydrate that is eaten to avoid postprandial hyperglycemia. Learning dietary skills is a difficult process for many children and parents and requires direct instruction and practice over time. Whereas carbohydrate counting is an important aid to attaining good glycemic control, it is also important for parents to be aware of low–glycemic index foods because flexible dietary regimens emphasizing these types of foods may improve glycemic control in children.

Children's activity levels also may vary considerably, raising the risk of either hypoglycemia or hyperglycemia, depending on baseline blood glucose, food consumed, and available insulin. It is important for children and parents to monitor blood glucose levels before, during, and after increased physical activity to avoid hypoglycemia or hyperglycemia. In addition, carrying short-acting carbohydrates is essential in treating hypoglycemia promptly. Because young children have frequent viral illnesses, parents need to know how to manage the effects of such illnesses on glycemic control.

Attaining and maintaining good glycemic control are of paramount importance, especially because the Diabetes Control and Complications Trial has established that "tight control" is associated with reduced health risks. However, during childhood, good control is often elusive. After repeated "trials," in which blood glucose levels seem unrelated to adherence to the prescribed regimen, parents and children may begin to feel that their self-care efforts are unrelated to glycemic outcomes. Eventually, these experiences may lead to a feeling of "learned helplessness," which has been associated with poor glycemic control in youths. Because learned helplessness may lead to depression and a feeling of "why bother to try?," it is important for children to talk about their experiences with their parents and the health care team, who can help them cope with their difficulties in adaptive ways (see Chapter 20).

New research has shown that intensive approaches to diabetes management, such as the use of continuous subcutaneous insulin infusion, not only lead to improved glycemic control, but also to reduced frequency of hypoglycemia and improved psychosocial adjustment and quality of life among youths. Parents and children should be encouraged that youth with diabetes can attain good control of their diabetes and work with their health care team over time to develop the skills and confidence necessary to achieve this goal. It is important for parents to use skillful approaches to facilitate increased self-care efforts in their children. Research has shown that an authoritative parenting style, characterized by warmth and structure, is related to better regimen adherence in children.

Help Parents Keep Tabs on Social Adjustment and Self-Esteem in Their Children

Self-esteem and social adjustment are significant psychosocial concerns related to daily diabetes management. Parents are often quite concerned with how their child will be accepted by peers. Older children are commonly concerned about being seen as different from other children because of what their diabetes regimen requires. Many parents and children may find it helpful to attend support groups with other families of children with diabetes.

KNOW WHEN TO INTERVENE

Parents and children have much to deal with at diagnosis. Although this is the time during which most diabetes education takes place, it is important to remember that anxiety interferes with learning. Everything that is taught may not be remembered. Think of education as a process that occurs over time. Experience helps to consolidate the concepts of diabetes care. Furthermore, remember that education does not necessarily lead to competencies with regimen-related skills and that having skills does not automatically lead to behavior change. Educate patients, teach them self-management skills, and help them succeed at changing their behavior.

At the time of diagnosis and during the first few weeks of adjustment, the child and family typically need a lot of psychological support. It is not unreasonable to consider this a crisis, requiring a crisis intervention approach. Reassure the family that their child can go on to live a happy life, that they will be able to learn to manage diabetes effectively, and that there is a team of health care professionals committed to helping them succeed.

After learning the most basic survival skills, the family is essentially on their own, with follow-up typically conducted at 2- to 3-month intervals and later at 3- to 4-month intervals. Because of the honeymoon phenomenon, fairly good glycemic control can be expected during the first 2 years or so after diagnosis. When residual β-cell activity dissipates, glycemic control may be more difficult to attain, and additional education and counseling may be required.

Rather than waiting for problems to develop, preventive approaches may be used before risk increases for problems with glycemic control. Two critical times for intervention are *1)* the period just after diagnosis and *2)* the period just before puberty.

KNOW HOW TO INTERVENE

There is evidence for the efficacy of behavioral interventions at the two critical times noted above. In one study, families who participated in self-management training during the first 4 months after diagnosis had children with significantly better glycemic control 2 years after diagnosis than patients who received conventional outpatient care without self-management training. In this study, self-management training focused on increasing the use of blood glucose monitoring for making behavioral changes to improve glycemic control. Specific home tests were prescribed to help patients and their families understand how food, exercise, and insulin affect blood glucose. The goal was to build family support for regimen adherence and to develop diabetes self-care strategies based on blood glucose measurements. The lessons from this study are as follows:

- provide education and behavioral interventions over a period of several months after diagnosis, before negative habits develop
- provide specific exercises so that families can experience for themselves how blood glucose is affected by various factors
- counsel parents to use positive reinforcement to encourage appropriate regimen behaviors in their children

In another study, a developmentally appropriate intervention was used that involved the peer group, practical applications of blood glucose monitoring, and parental counseling to establish reasonable self-care responsibilities and parental involvement. The intervention was administered at the clinic in a group format, with separate groups for children and parents. Children who received this intervention had better glycemic control over an 18-month period than those treated conventionally.

Much can be applied from the extensive literature on psychological interventions for children's behavioral disorders and regimen noncompliance. Many controlled studies have demonstrated the effectiveness of parent training in effective child behavior management strategies to reduce noncompliant behaviors in children. In general, parents tend to ignore positive behaviors and attend to and inadvertently reinforce negative behaviors. Essentially, brief interventions (six to eight sessions) focus on teaching parents to differentially reinforce their children's behavior: appropriate compliant behavior is positively reinforced, minor negative behavior is ignored (extinguished), and more serious noncompliant behavior is punished (using the "time-out" technique or loss of privileges). In addition, instructions in giving commands or making requests are provided because noncompliance in children is often associated with ineffective methods of command-giving in parents. Token economies and behavioral contracts may be used successfully to improve behaviors such as those involved in the diabetes regimen. In a token economy, specific target behaviors are rewarded with points or tokens that can be exchanged later for desired reinforcers. Behavioral contracts specify the child's responsibilities and the privileges earned contingent upon completion of tasks.

It is important that parents of children with diabetes be instructed in effective behavior management techniques: give clear expectations, apply positive reinforcement for successful performance with the regimen, and administer consistent consequences for nonadherence. These approaches have been used successfully in a number of controlled studies of youths with diabetes. In particular, interventions using goal-setting, memos, self-monitoring or charting, behavioral contracts, and social problem-solving with behavioral rehearsal have been effective in improving adherence to various components of the regimen, and sometimes in improving glycemic control as well. It is important to help older children understand which social situations are associated with adherence problems, identify appropriate strategies for prevention of these problems, and rehearse with them how to implement those strategies. Successful interventions have been conducted with individual families and also with groups of children and parents. Recent studies have shown that family-based interventions to improve parent-adolescent teamwork, parental support, and family communication have resulted in improvements in regimen adherence, glycemic control, and parent-adolescent relationships. In addition, coping skills training has been shown to improve glycemic control as well as quality of life in youths.

CONCLUSION

Successful management of diabetes in young children presents significant challenges for all involved—parents, children, and the health care team. Whereas optimal glycemic control is desired, it is critical that reasonable goals be established, with consideration given to the changing regimen requirements related to the process of development in the growing child. Success should be measured not only by glycemic outcomes, but also by attainment of age-appropriate regimen-related skills and responsibilities, as well as emotional, social, and academic development. Because diabetes management in children occurs within a family context, attention must be given to family functioning. Many studies have shown its importance in relation to health behaviors and metabolic outcomes. Encourage parents to find ways to be supportive of their child's self-care efforts while minimizing the use of nonsupportive strategies such as criticizing, nagging, and arguing (see Chapter 19).

Early interventions may prevent later problems with regimen adherence and metabolic control. The months after diagnosis are an optimal time to lay the groundwork for successful self-management. Counsel parents about the importance of positive reinforcement for performance of appropriate regimen-related behaviors. Involvement of children in performing self-care behaviors can begin in early childhood, but responsibilities for these tasks must be developmentally appropriate. Treatment should include the cultivation of adaptive thinking about and coping with less than optimal glycemic outcomes because feelings of helplessness may adversely affect later performance of health behaviors.

Be responsive to the needs of the family, particularly in the period after diagnosis, but also throughout the course of the child's development, when the needs of the child and family may not be consistent with the prescriptions offered by the team. It is essential for normal development to proceed unhindered by the demands of diabetes management. When the two become intertwined, problems will arise.

Pay attention to family conflict, poor communication between parents and children, isolation of the family from social supports, high levels of parental stress, and difficulties with children's school performance and psychosocial adjustment. Clearly, these problems and difficulties with regimen adherence and glycemic control may indicate the need for referral to a mental health professional who is knowledgeable about diabetes and its management in children.

Many of the guidelines offered here for behavioral interventions are simple but not easy. Behavioral changes are often gradual rather than sudden and dramatic. Patience and encouragement are essential, along with reasonable expectations for success and demonstrations by the health care team of interest and commitment to the patient and family (see Chapter 3). The principles of reinforcement are thus as applicable and important from the health care team to the family as from the parents to the child.

BIBLIOGRAPHY

Anderson BJ, Brackett J, Ho J, Laffel LMB: An office-based intervention to maintain parent-adolescent teamwork in diabetes management: impact on parent involvement, family conflict, and subsequent glycemic control. *Diabetes Care* 22:713–721, 1999

Anderson BJ, Wolf RM, Burkhart MT, Cornell RG, Bacon GE: Effects of peer-group intervention on metabolic control of adolescents with IDDM: randomized outpatient study. *Diabetes Care* 12:179–183, 1989

Auslander WF, Thompson S, Dreitzer D, White NH, Santiago JV: Disparity in glycemic control and adherence between African American and Caucasian youths with diabetes: family and community contexts. *Diabetes Care* 20:1569–1575, 1997

Barkley RA: *Defiant Children: A Clinician's Manual for Parent Training.* New York, Guilford Press, 1987

Boland EA, Grey M, Oesterle A, Fredrickson L, Tamborlane WV: Continuous subcutaneous insulin infusion: a new way to lower risk of severe hypoglycemia, improve metabolic control, and enhance coping in adolescents with type 1 diabetes. *Diabetes Care* 22:1779–1784, 1999

Davis CL, Delamater AM, Shaw, KH, La Greca AM, Eidson M, Perez-Rodriguez J, Nemery R: Parenting styles, regimen adherence, and glycemic control in 4- to 10-year-old children with diabetes. *J Pediatr Psychol* 26:123–129, 2001

Delamater AM, Bubb J, Davis SG, Smith JA, Schmidt L, White NH, Santiago JV: Randomized prospective study of self-management training with newly diagnosed diabetic children. *Diabetes Care* 13:492–498, 1990

Delamater AM, Jacobson AM, Anderson BJ, Cox D, Fisher L, Lustman P, Rubin R, Wysocki T: Psychosocial therapies in diabetes: report of the Psychosocial Therapies Working Group. *Diabetes Care* 24:1286–1292, 2001

Delamater AM, Shaw K, Applegate EB, Pratt IA, Eidson M, Lancelotta G, Gonzalez-Mendoza L, Richton S: Risk for metabolic control problems in minority youth with diabetes. *Diabetes Care* 22:700–705, 1999

Gilbertson HR, Grand-Miller JC, Thorburn AW, Evans S, Chondros P, Werther GA: The effect of flexible low glycemic index dietary advice versus measured carbohydrate exchange diets on glycemic control in children with type 1 diabetes. *Diabetes Care* 24:1137–1143, 2001

Grey M, Boland EA, Davidson M, Yu C, Sullivan-Bolyai S, Tamborlane WV: Short-term effects of coping skills training as adjunct to intensive therapy in adolescents. *Diabetes Care* 21:902–908, 1998

Johnson SB: Insulin-dependent diabetes mellitus in childhood. In *Handbook of Pediatric Psychology.* 2nd ed. Roberts M, Ed. New York, Guilford Press, 1995, pp. 263–285

Marteau TM, Johnson M, Baum JD, Bloch S: Goals of treatment in diabetes: comparison of doctors and parents of children with diabetes. *J Behav Med* 10:33–48, 1987

Miller-Johnson S, Emery RE, Marvin RS, Clarke W, Lovinger R, Martin M: Parent-child relationships and the management of insulin-dependent diabetes mellitus. *J Consult Clin Psychol* 62:603–610, 1994

Northam EA, Anderson PJ, Jacobs R, Hughes M, Warne GL, Werther GA: Neuropsychological profiles of children with type 1 diabetes 6 years after disease onset. *Diabetes Care* 24:1541–1546, 2001

Satin W, La Grecfa A, Zigo M, Skyler J: Diabetes in adolescence: effects of multifamily group intervention and parent simulation of diabetes. *J Pediatr Psychol* 14:259–276, 1989

Wysocki T, Greco P, Harris MA, Bubb J, White NH: Behavior therapy for families of adolescents with diabetes. *Diabetes Care* 24:441–446, 2001

Wysocki T, Meinhold PA, Abrams KC, Barnard MU, Clarke WL, Bellando BJ, Bourgeois MJ: Parental and professional estimates of self-care independence of children and adolescents with IDDM. *Diabetes Care* 15:43–52, 1992

Wysocki T, Taylor A, Hough B, Linscheid T, Yeates K, Naglieri J: Deviation from developmentally appropriate self-care autonomy: association with diabetes outcomes. *Diabetes Care* 19:119–125, 1996

Alan M. Delamater, PhD, ABPP, is a Professor of Pediatrics and Psychology at the University of Miami School of Medicine in Miami, FL.

13

Working with Adolescents

RICHARD R. RUBIN, PhD, CDE

Adolescence is filled with joys and woes under any circumstances. This transition is complicated in myriad ways—large and small—by diabetes. The dramatic changes of adolescence often distract a young person from diabetes self-care, and the normal hormonal changes of adolescence also contribute to variable blood glucose levels and elevated glycated hemoglobin A1C (A1C) levels.

This developmental stage presents the health care provider with a challenge and an opportunity. The opportunity lies in the adolescent's countless (though often unexpressed) specific concerns about living with diabetes. These concerns represent powerful "teachable moments": opportunities to help adolescents make diabetes care more effective or easier. The health care provider who is able to identify and address these concerns will see striking improvements in a range of diabetes outcomes. This chapter contains guidelines for helping clinicians work with adolescents who have diabetes.

BE CLEAR ABOUT THE ROLES ADOLESCENTS, PARENTS, AND HEALTH CARE PROVIDERS PLAY IN DIABETES CARE

All parties involved in diabetes care should be clear about their roles. The health care provider's role is to help the adolescent learn to manage his or her diabetes. The parent's role is similar. The adolescent's role is to work collaboratively with the health care provider and his or her parents. This collaboration has to respect some basic principles if it is going to work.

Principles of Collaborative Diabetes Care

- Adolescents control diabetes care. They are the chief executive officers of their diabetes team. They make the vast majority of clinically relevant diabetes care decisions and make these decisions—about eating, medication taking, activity, and blood glucose monitoring—countless times each day. These countless decisions, some made wisely and some made with no thought whatsoever, all affect health outcomes.
- Adolescents' diabetes care decisions reflect the unique reality of *their* lives with diabetes, including the pressure of competing priorities; the support they get from family, friends, teachers, and health care providers; how mature they are; and how good their coping skills are.
- Though it may often appear otherwise to adults, all adolescents want to be healthy; most feel uncomfortable when their blood glucose levels are low or very high, and all want to avoid complications.
- All adolescents are motivated to actively manage their diabetes when they see the benefit and see that active management is not too inconvenient (see Chapter 15).
- Adolescents need to be more independent; therefore, they are often less willing to do what adults (including parents and health care providers) tell them to do. Adolescents also need to find out who they really are, so they may become passionately engaged in a variety of new interests and activities, leaving less time and energy for the often-burdensome routine of diabetes care.
- Parents and health care providers have special expertise and resources to help make diabetes management easier and more effective.
- Adolescents welcome help with diabetes management when the personal benefits are clear and the burden bearable.
- When diabetes care is truly collaborative, adolescents get the help they need from health care providers and parents to solve the diabetes-related problems that bother them most, and they use this help to build skill in managing diabetes independently.

ADDRESS THE ADOLESCENT'S AGENDA FIRST

Starting with the adolescent's concerns is essential. This reinforces the roles of all parties in diabetes care, it facilitates change by addressing first the issues the adolescent is most highly motivated to address, and it helps the adolescent learn general problem-solving skills to apply to new situations.

Asking questions such as, "What is the hardest thing for you right now about living with diabetes?" or "What one thing about dealing with diabetes would you most like to change?" can help identify issues to address (see Chapter 6). Often these concerns will be diabetes-specific expressions of normal developmental issues. For example:

- Am I physically attractive? ("Insulin makes me gain weight, I have lumps at injection sites, my fingers look ugly where I stick them for blood tests.")
- Do I fit in? ("I feel uncomfortable stopping to take shots or do blood tests and having to eat the right thing at the right time.")
- Is there something wrong with me? ("Going low, carrying supplies, testing blood, and taking shots are so embarrassing.")
- Can I do what I want? ("I can't eat, drink, and stay up late like other kids.")
- Am I ready to be on my own? ("Can I manage my diabetes independently?")

Once identified, diabetes-related concerns represent "teachable moments" when the health care provider can help the young person make wise diabetes care decisions. Often these decisions involve more physiological insulin replacement, to maximize flexibility and minimize weight gain and risk of hypoglycemia. These decisions, driven by the adolescent's desire to make diabetes care easier or more effective, will often improve both glycemic control and quality of life.

ENCOURAGE POSITIVE INVOLVEMENT

Most adolescents welcome adult involvement in diabetes care when it feels like support and not pushing. Involvement is supportive when it helps a person do something he or she wants to do (see above) and when it is delivered in a positive tone at an appropriate time. One young woman was having trouble remembering to monitor her blood glucose before dinner. Her mother agreed to help by asking her if she had tested each evening before they sat down to eat. Halfway through dinner the next evening, the mother suddenly remembered her assignment and angrily blurted, "You didn't test, did you?" Fortunately, the mother quickly recognized that her tone and timing left something to be desired. She apologized for her approach and asked the question *before* dinner and more pleasantly from then on.

Focusing on successes also makes adult involvement in diabetes care more positive. "Catching" adolescents when they are good and talking about it reinforces self-confidence and motivation for self-care. Whenever a typically problematic situation is less troublesome, compliments are in order. Trying to pinpoint what helped the situation go more smoothly can also be useful. Starting with compliments may make the young person more receptive to this process. Research confirms that parental involvement in diabetes management can be beneficial, but only under certain circumstances. The key to success seems to be *teamwork*, with responsibilities clearly defined and with little *overlap*. One study found that family conflict was lowest when parents and adolescents were both involved in diabetes management, but only when each party was responsible for different tasks. When parents were involved in tasks for which the adolescents felt responsible, conflict was higher.

Parent-adolescent teamwork can be fostered by open discussions of who is responsible for what when it comes to diabetes care. These discussions should respect all the principles of collaborative care noted earlier in this chapter. A variety of interventions, including clinic-based education and training programs and brief family therapy, have been shown to improve parent-adolescent teamwork in diabetes management. This teamwork has a range of positive consequences, including more family harmony, more active diabetes care, and better glycemic control in the adolescents.

MAKE SURE BLOOD GLUCOSE GOALS ARE REALISTIC

Perfect blood glucose control is an impossible dream. The intensive treatment group of the Diabetes Control and Complications Trial (DCCT), who were highly motivated and had state-of-the-art professional care, were unable, as a group, to achieve normoglycemia. In fact, only 20% of the entire group ever achieved a normal A1C reading during the course of the trial, and only 5% maintained normal A1C levels throughout the study. Among the teenagers who participated in the DCCT, the proportion who achieved normal A1C levels was even lower.

As difficult as it is to achieve at any age, normoglycemia is probably uniquely unachievable during adolescence (see Chapter 14). The physiological changes of this period, which are associated with insulin resistance in both diabetic and nondiabetic teenagers, contribute to blood glucose instability. Combined with the need to test one's wings, which often means less attention to diabetes care, blood glucose control during adolescence is often particularly rocky.

Pushing adolescents and their parents to achieve blood glucose goals that are beyond their reach can actually contribute to poorer glycemic control; feelings of hopelessness may reduce motivation for self-care (see Chapter 21). Helping families set more realistic goals, including a step-by-step approach to getting blood glucose levels as close to normal as possible, fosters self-confidence, enhances motivation for self-care, and improves long-term health.

DO NOT ENCOURAGE INDEPENDENT CARE BASED ON AGE ALONE

Until about 15 years ago, there was strong support for getting children to manage their own diabetes care as quickly as possible. Independent diabetes care was seen as a sign of maturity or responsibility. But now it is clear that parental involvement in diabetes care can be a good thing, regardless of the child's age. Recent research found that the more involved parents were in their children's diabetes management, the lower the child's A1C level.

People of any age appreciate help and support with diabetes care, at least from time to time. Adolescents certainly continue to need this help. Keep in mind that there is almost always a big difference between a teenager's *physical* capacity to master a task and the *cognitive* and *emotional* maturity required to carry out the task on a continuing basis. One study found that when parents turned over diabetes management tasks to their children, the adolescents often did not always take them over; tasks such as insulin adjustment often went undone.

Guidelines for independent self-care should also take into account an adolescent's individual circumstances, including temperament, special strengths and challenges, and family resources and problems. Regular reevaluation of the adolescent's diabetes self-care skills and the family's division of diabetes tasks should guide recommendations for shifting diabetes care responsibility to the adolescent.

HELP TEENS AND THEIR PARENTS DEAL WITH FEELINGS

Living with diabetes makes life more stressful; therefore, patients and their parents are bound to feel frustrated, scared, and angry, at least occasionally. When they do, they need a constructive way to deal with these feelings. Helping families focus their anger (or other upset feelings) on the diabetes—rather than on each other—puts teens and their parents on the same side of the fence. This scenario can dramatically reduce family conflict and enhance the potential for collaborative diabetes care.

Providers and parents often find it hard to hear a teen express strong negative feelings about diabetes because they do not know what to do about the feelings. They want to "fix" the feelings, to somehow protect the adolescent from the pain. But the best thing any caring adult can do—in fact, the *only* helpful thing to do—is to listen to the adolescent and to sympathize. Feeling bad about diabetes is natural, normal, and even inevitable (see Chapter 20). Teens who know their health care providers and parents understand this are much more likely to welcome a collaborative approach to managing their diabetes.

HELP THE ADOLESCENT BUILD COPING SKILLS

Adolescents need two sets of skills to live well with diabetes: *1*) specific *self-care* skills, such as knowing how to monitor blood glucose levels and adjust food and insulin, and *2*) diabetes-specific *coping* skills, such as being able to deal with the stress and emotional challenges of managing diabetes effectively in real-life situations (e.g., at parties). Research shows that coping skills matter: adolescents who effectively cope also tend to monitor blood glucose more often, eat more carefully, and adjust insulin doses more often. Adolescents can learn diabetes-specific coping skills. One intervention taught adolescents how to cope better with potentially challenging diabetes-related social situations by using role-playing, and cognitive restructuring and conflict resolution techniques. Adolescents who participated in this intervention had lower A1C levels and improved quality of life 6 months after the intervention compared with adolescents in the study's control group. In other studies, coping skills training helped young people feel more confident about managing their diabetes and helped them cope better with the demands of diabetes management. For more on diabetes coping skills, see Chapter 6.

NOURISH HOPE AND HUMOR

Hope is a barrier against the stresses and strains of life with diabetes. And faith in oneself is a wonderful source of hope and optimism. A 15-year-old boy sat with his father talking about things they wished for. When his father said he wished his son didn't have diabetes, the boy said, "I don't wish that. It's not that I like diabetes; in fact, I hate it. But having diabetes has forced me to learn how to take care of myself. I can take care of myself better than any of my friends, and I wouldn't give that up for anything in the world." When we nourish adolescents' faith in themselves, they gain one of life's most precious gifts. This faith will help them live well with their diabetes and with other life challenges. Help patients think of things from which they draw comfort or inspiration.

Humor is also powerful. Many daily diabetes dilemmas have a funny side when seen from the right perspective. One Thanksgiving evening some years ago, a family's holiday anticipation was disrupted by a crisis: the teenage son's insulin pump had stopped working, and nothing he or his dad could think of got it working again. It looked like something was stuck in the drive that pushed the insulin out of the reservoir. The young man prevailed upon his father—who was no handyman—to use some pliers and free the drive. Six months earlier when the boy got his pump, he swore he would never take another shot. He had no intentions of going back on that vow. So very much against his better judgement, the father tried, and he miraculously succeeded in fixing the pump. Once the ordeal was over, the young man looked over at his father and said, "You sure are lucky." Then laughing, he added, "You would not want to spend a holiday weekend with me if my pump wasn't working." His father laughed too, and the tension washed away. Humor can be an important source of strength and comfort, relieving stress and helping keep self-care on track.

ADDRESS SERIOUS PSYCHOLOGICAL PROBLEMS

Some psychological disorders, including depression and adjustment disorders, seem to be more common among adolescents with diabetes than among their peers who do not have diabetes. Health care providers should identify patients who may be suffering from psychological disorders and refer them for diagnosis and treatment; depression and other psychological problems severely compromise physical and emotional well-being in adolescents with diabetes. Adolescents who are depressed may find it nearly impossible to maintain active self-care, thus dramatically increasing the risk for acute and chronic complications. Studies show that resolving depression in people with diabetes also generally improves glycemic control. Special care should be taken to identify young people who may be at risk for suicide.

Adolescents who suffer from an anxiety disorder may be so concerned about the possibility of becoming hypoglycemic that they purposely keep blood glucose levels very high. Eating disorders may be more common among young people with diabetes (see Chapter 23), and there is no doubt that these disorders have more devastating effects when the person has diabetes because metabolic control can be so severely compromised.

A positive, consistent bond with the adolescent patient helps the health care provider identify possible psychological disorders. This bond can also facilitate successful referral of the young person to a mental health professional for further evaluation and treatment, when it is indicated. Referral to someone who has experience treating people with diabetes is highly recommended. For more on recognizing and treating depression in people with diabetes, see Chapter 22.

MAINTAIN CONTACT

It is important to regularly check in with adolescent patients between visits to see how they are doing. This can be difficult, given the busy schedules most clinicians maintain, but any contact between appointments can be helpful. Each time the teenager comes in, ask about any new problems that might have come up and about any successes the patient has had managing his or her diabetes. When time is limited, try to focus on whatever issue is of greatest concern to the adolescent (see Chapter 1).

It is also essential that patients' parents do all they can to maintain contact with their children. Some families have regularly scheduled diabetes family meetings when everyone gets to say anything about how things have been going since the last meeting. This can be a good opportunity to deal with small problems before they become big ones. The key to success with these meetings is maintaining an attitude of cooperation and collaboration.

CONCLUSION

Working with adolescents who have diabetes can be uniquely challenging. But if clinicians work wisely with patients and their parents, facilitating the process by which young people learn to manage their disease, this work can be uniquely rewarding as well.

BIBLIOGRAPHY

Anderson BJ, Brackett J, Ho J, Laffel LMB: An office-based intervention to maintain parent-adolescent teamwork in diabetes management: impact on parental involvement, family conflict, and subsequent glycemic control. *Diabetes Care* 22:713–721, 1999

Brackenridge BP, Rubin RR: *Sweet Kids: How to Balance Diabetes Control and Good Nutrition With Family Peace.* 2nd ed. Alexandria, VA, American Diabetes Association, 2002

Grey M, Boland EA, Davidson M, Yu C, Sullivan-Bolyai S, Tamborlane WV: Short-term effects of coping skills training as adjunct to intensive therapy in adolescents. *Diabetes Care* 21:902–908, 1998

Rubin RR, Biermann J, Toohey B: *Psyching Out Diabetes.* Los Angeles, CA, Lowell House, 1992

Wolpert HA, Anderson BJ: The young adult with diabetes: need for a new treatment paradigm. *Diabetes Care* 24:1513–1514, 2001

Wysocki T, Greco P, Harris MA, Bubb J, White NH: Behavior therapy for families of adolescents with diabetes: maintenance of treatment effects. *Diabetes Care* 24:441–446, 2001

Wysocki T, Taylor A, Hough B, Linscheid T, Yeates K, Naglieri J: Deviation from developmentally appropriate self-care autonomy. *Diabetes Care* 19:119–125, 1996

Richard R. Rubin, PhD, CDE, is an Associate Professor of Medicine and Pediatrics at The Johns Hopkins University School of Medicine in Baltimore, MD.

14

Improving Diabetes Control in Adolescents with Type 1 Diabetes

JOSEPH I. WOLFSDORF, MB, BCH

Optimal treatment during puberty is necessary to ensure normal growth and physical development and to prevent, slow, or reverse the progression of diabetic microvascular complications. The landmark Diabetes Control and Complications Trial (DCCT) demonstrated that the beneficial effects of intensive therapy in adolescents were similar to those observed in adults. In a recent Swedish population study, the incidence of diabetic nephropathy after 25 years, in patients in whom diabetes was diagnosed before age 15 years, declined as a result of improved glycemic control. Therapy should aim to maintain blood glucose levels as near to normal as possible and to lower glycated hemoglobin A1C (A1C) to achieve maximum prevention of complications with due regard for patient safety. Intensive management is required to achieve this goal. Developmental considerations and the endocrinologic effects of puberty make this a daunting task (see Chapter 13).

UNDERSTAND LESSONS FROM THE DCCT

Of the 1,441 subjects who participated in the DCCT, 13.5% were adolescents (13–17 years old at the time of enrollment) who were followed for a mean of 7.4 years. At baseline, the mean A1C in the adolescent cohort was ~9.5% (upper limit of normal is 6.05%), whereas the adult cohort started with a mean A1C of ~8.5%. With the institution of intensive diabetes therapy, mean A1C levels of both the adult and adolescent cohorts decreased by about 2 percentage points. By the end of the first year of the study, it was evident that the adolescent cohort was unable to lower blood glucose and A1C to the level achieved by the adult cohort. This difference between adolescents and adults persisted even in this select population who received free and unlimited access to an expert diabetes care team. Less than 2% of adolescents maintained A1C levels ≤6.05%, and only 29% were able to achieve the target of ≤6.05% at least once in the course of the study. Mean A1C levels of adolescents are compared with those of adults in Table 14.1. Expectations for A1C levels for adolescent patients must reflect these realistic limitations.

RECOGNIZE ADOLESCENT DEVELOPMENTAL CONSIDERATIONS

Treatment of type 1 diabetes in children and adolescents occurs on a background of physical, cognitive, and emotional growth and development. Until maturity is attained, developmental issues influence the health care team's efforts to manage diabetes (see Chapter 15). Despite the challenges, the diabetes clinician should patiently, but persistently, help the patient to manage his or her diabetes as well as possible, mindful of the fact that the goals of therapy currently may not be reached in an individual patient.

RECOGNIZE THE ENDOCRINOLOGIC EFFECTS OF PUBERTY

Glycemic control often deteriorates with the onset of puberty. This deterioration is often attributed to adolescents' poor compliance with diet and insulin administration. But behavioral and psychosocial issues are not the only factors that affect blood glucose control during this stage of development. Endocrinologic changes of puberty significantly contribute to the deterioration in glycemic control.

- Insulin resistance normally occurs during puberty and contributes to the difficulty of achieving optimal glycemic control during ado-

TABLE 14.1 Mean A1C Levels of Adolescents Compared With Adults in the DCCT

	Adolescents (%)	Adults (%)
Intensive	8.06 ± 0.13	7.12 ± 0.03
Conventional	9.76 ± 0.12	9.02 ± 0.05
Difference (intensive vs. conventional)	1.70 ± 0.18	1.90 ± 0.06

Data are means ± SE. Adapted from Diabetes Control and Complications Research Group: Effect of intensive diabetes treatment on the development and progression of long-term complications in adolescents with insulin-dependent diabetes mellitus: Diabetes Control and Complications Trial. *J Pediatr* 125:177–188, 1994.

lescence. During puberty, physiological insulin resistance results in an increase in daily insulin requirement by ≥50%.

- Diurnal variation in insulin requirements, which reach a nadir between midnight and 3:00 A.M. and increase from 5:00 to 9:00 A.M. (the dawn phenomenon), is typically more pronounced during puberty, making overnight insulin replacement even more challenging.

- During the period of accelerated growth characteristic of puberty, both nutritional and insulin requirements markedly increase. To ensure the best possible metabolic control, schedule follow-up visits for medical supervision at least once every 3 months until completion of growth. Regular visits with the diabetes clinician provide an opportunity to review self-monitoring of blood glucose (SMBG) data, measure A1C, and determine if insulin doses need to be adjusted or the regimen altered to match the youth's lifestyle.

HELP ADOLESCENTS TO USE A MORE PHYSIOLOGICAL INSULIN REPLACEMENT REGIMEN

Many adolescents are willing to accept an insulin replacement regimen that involves more frequent insulin administration (either with a syringe or an insulin pen device), which permits greater flexibility of meal times and lifestyle. Continuous subcutaneous insulin infusion (CSII), or pump therapy, is an appropriate option for some adolescents and can effectively decrease A1C and the frequency of severe hypoglycemic episodes without leading to excessive weight gain. Successful use of any multiple-dose regimen or CSII requires considerable self-management training to enable the youth to interpret SMBG data, to adjust timing of insulin administration and doses, and to make appropriate food selections. **The goal is to equip the adolescent patient with problem-solving skills to cope with unexpected situations and unplanned events typical of the adolescent lifestyle** (see Chapter 6), for example, additional, late, or omitted meals; "pickup" games; travel to events away from home; participation in competitive sports; and variable sleep times.

- After the honeymoon or remission period, which frequently begins soon after diagnosis and extends for 3–12 months or longer, optimal delivery of insulin requires use of a physiological insulin replacement regimen, either with multiple doses of insulin (MDI) or CSII.

- If an adolescent patient is not already using an MDI regimen, encourage him or her to use at least a three-dose regimen: a mixed dose (rapid- or short- and intermediate-acting insulins) before breakfast, rapid- or short-acting insulin before the evening meal, and intermediate-acting insulin (with or without rapid-acting insulin) before bedtime.

- Regimens in which intermediate-acting insulin is given before the evening meal do not provide optimal overnight insulin delivery. Too much insulin is provided between 11:00 P.M. and 4:00 A.M., which may cause symptomatic or asymptomatic hypoglycemia, whereas waning insulin action before breakfast results in high pre- and post-breakfast blood glucose concentrations. An intermediate-acting insulin (NPH or lente) given at bedtime will provide the increased insulin required before breakfast and reduce the risk of hypoglycemia between 11:00 P.M. and 4:00 A.M. The long-acting, peakless insulin analog glargine is a recently available alternative method to lower pre-breakfast blood glucose levels and decrease the risk of nocturnal hypoglycemia. The variable basal rate feature of insulin pumps is especially useful to facilitate optimal overnight insulin delivery in youth with a pronounced dawn phenomenon.

- A dose of rapid-acting insulin before lunch and/or before a large after-school snack is the best method to prevent hyperglycemia in the late afternoon. This is not always necessary, and, for the youth unwilling to use a four-dose regimen, a mixed dose of insulin before breakfast may achieve excellent blood glucose control in the afternoon, provided that the carbohydrate content of lunch and the afternoon snack is not excessive.

LEARN TO MATCH FOOD WITH INSULIN

Attention must be paid to the timing and content of meals and snacks to match food intake with the availability of injected insulin.

- The aim of nutritional counseling is to encourage the patient to use a meal plan that fits his or her lifestyle, promotes optimal adherence, and advances the goals of management.
- In the DCCT, adherence to a meal plan and adjusting food and/or insulin in response to hyperglycemia was associated with significantly lower (0.25–1.0%) levels of A1C. Adjusting the insulin dose for meal size and carbohydrate content and consistent consumption of an evening snack were also associated with lower levels of A1C. These findings underscore the importance of nutritional counseling to enhance the patient's ability to match insulin availability to food consumption.
- From the time of diagnosis, teach the patient the principles of nutritional management of diabetes, and individualize the meal plan to minimize postprandial hyperglycemia and hypoglycemia between meals.
- Teach patients how to use supplemental rapid-acting insulin to correct high blood glucose levels before meals and how to treat hypoglycemia without causing post-hypoglycemic hyperglycemia.
- The process of nutrition education should be staged, i.e., begin with "survival" information using food exchanges and gradually progress to more advanced topics: counting carbohydrates, reading food labels, adjusting insulin dose for carbohydrate content of meals, and managing eating away from home (see Chapter 7).

ENCOURAGE REGULAR EXERCISE

- Encourage teenagers with diabetes to participate in sports and to exercise regularly throughout the year. In addition to normalizing the adolescent's life and helping to form a positive self-image, exercise promotes good health practices, facilitates weight control, and may improve glycemic control by decreasing the physiological insulin resistance of puberty. Adolescents with type 1 diabetes who maintain a high level of physical fitness are relatively less insulin resistant.

- Exercise acutely lowers blood glucose concentrations by increasing the rate of glucose utilization, which depends on the intensity and duration of physical activity and the concurrent serum level of insulin. Teach teenagers strategies to prevent exercise-related hypoglycemia (see Chapter 8). Ideally, when starting a new exercise program, have teenagers measure blood glucose before, during, and after exercise so that rational adjustments can be made to the insulin dose, meals, and snacks.

- In the absence of SMBG data, have teenagers cover unplanned physical activity with a snack before and, if the exercise is prolonged, during the activity. A useful rule of thumb is to provide 15 g carbohydrate (one Starch or Fruit exchange) for every 30–60 min of vigorous physical activity.

- Advise youth who participate in organized sports to reduce the dose of the insulin that is most active during the period of sustained physical activity. The precise amount of such reductions has to be determined by measuring blood glucose levels before and after exercise. These reductions are generally in the range of 10–30% of the usual insulin dose.

- Exercising the limb into which insulin has been injected accelerates its rate of absorption; therefore, have patients give the insulin injection preceding planned exercise in a site where absorption is least likely to be affected by exercise.

- After strenuous exercise in the afternoon or evening, advise patients to reduce the presupper and/or bedtime dose of intermediate-acting insulin by 10–20% and to eat a larger bedtime snack, to reduce the risk of nocturnal or early-morning hypoglycemia (lag effect of exercise).

- Make sure the youth is aware that ketonuria is a reason to **not** exercise because acute vigorous exercise under these circumstances can aggravate hyperglycemia and ketoacid production.

RECOGNIZE THAT BLOOD GLUCOSE MONITORING IS THE CORNERSTONE OF INTENSIVE DIABETES MANAGEMENT

- Encourage patients to measure blood glucose levels at least before each meal and at bedtime. Because of discomfort and inconvenience, many adolescents are unwilling to perform frequent finger sticks. Encourage them to use alternative site testing. If the patient is unwilling or unable to monitor at least four times daily, negotiate blood glucose measurements before each dose of insulin and before lunch and at bedtime at least twice each week. For patients who simply refuse to perform regular SMBG, a period of intensive monitoring (before each meal, at bedtime, and between 2:00 and 4:00 A.M.) for several consecutive days before an office visit may provide sufficient information to reveal a blood glucose pattern that suggests simple modifications of the insulin regimen. Obviously, intensive diabetes management cannot be practiced in such a patient.

- Teenagers may fabricate blood glucose measurements because of pressure from their family members and physicians to produce "good" results. This behavior can be minimized if parents and physician avoid being judgmental when reviewing SMBG data with the patient (see Chapter 13). Clinicians should convey the notion that blood glucose levels are in the target range, high, or low, not "good" or "bad."

- Instructing patients to measure blood glucose levels without teaching them how to interpret the data is unlikely to improve diabetes control. The data should be reviewed and analyzed with the patient. The encounter is an opportunity to educate the patient in self-management skills. These skills include, but are not limited to, the following: how to analyze and interpret the numbers, how to use insulin dosage algorithms to select and adjust doses, how to make appropriate food choices, and how to plan exercise.

- Frequent SMBG is also essential to manage intercurrent illness and prevent ketoacidosis. Have patients test their urine or blood ketones whenever sick and when the level of blood glucose exceeds 250 mg/dl.

- Measure A1C every 3 months to provide a measure of average glycemia in the intervals between office visits and involve the patient in setting his or her A1C target.

ESTABLISH BIOCHEMICAL GOALS OF THERAPY

The goal of treatment is to maintain blood glucose levels as close to normal (80–120 mg/dl before meals and <180 mg/dl 90–120 min after meals) while minimizing the occurrence of hypoglycemia. The DCCT found that any reduction in A1C level was rewarded by a reduction in the risk of microvascular complications. The DCCT and other studies of adolescents have also demonstrated that, even with intensive methods of treatment, access to expert medical care and advice, and supervision by a specialist diabetes team, it is extremely difficult to achieve the goal of near-normal A1C levels in adolescents with type 1 diabetes.

PREVENT HYPOGLYCEMIA

Hypoglycemia is the principal adverse effect of intensive diabetes management and can be a major obstacle to achieving and maintaining tight glycemic control. Fear of hypoglycemia is an important determinant (often unstated) of patients' personal goals for glycemic control. In the DCCT, both intensively managed adults and adolescents had three times as many episodes of severe hypoglycemia as their conventionally treated peers. The overall incidence of severe hypoglycemia was even higher in adolescents than in adults: 86 vs. 57 events per 100 patient-years. In the ABCs (**A**dolescents **B**enefit from **C**ontrol) of Diabetes Study, severe hypoglycemia was less frequent with treatment by CSII than MDI (76 vs. 134 events per 100 patient-years). Others have reported that desirable glycemic control can be achieved without increasing the frequency and severity of hypoglycemia. Despite the increased risk of hypoglycemia, the reduction in risk of microvascular and neurological complications in adolescents outweighs the increased risk of severe hypoglycemia.

Be mindful of adolescent patients' vulnerability to hypoglycemia. Teach patients how to anticipate and prevent hypoglycemia and to treat it promptly without causing hyperglycemia. Begin treatment with 15 g glucose (preferably in the form of glucose tablets), and repeat the dose if the blood glucose level has not risen after 20 min. Practical guidelines for reducing the risk of hypoglycemia appear in Chapter 11.

SHARE RESPONSIBILITY FOR DIABETES CARE

Cognitive Maturity

The ability of an adolescent with type 1 diabetes to successfully assume primary responsibility for his or her diabetes care is related to age, duration of diabetes, and the individual's level of cognitive maturity. Intensive management of type 1 diabetes requires considerable patient participation in self-care and day-to-day decision-making. Indeed, the patient with diabetes has to learn to become his or her own health care provider.

Technical mastery of self-care skills and a thorough knowledge of the disease and its treatment are essential to assuming this role. The willingness and ability to perform the numerous tasks required to safely achieve desirable blood glucose control depend, substantially, on the individual's level of cognitive maturity. Age alone must not determine the appropriate time to transfer responsibility for self-care from parents to their adolescent child. The process of transfer should be gradual, accomplished over years, with decreasing parental supervision as adolescents consistently demonstrate the ability to care competently for themselves without deterioration of blood glucose control. Deterioration in glycemic control is less likely to occur and can be minimized when parents remain actively involved in their young adolescent child's diabetes care.

Family Functioning

Adolescents depend on their parents for material as well as emotional support and guidance. The functioning of the family system, therefore, has a major influence on the adolescent patient's diabetes care behavior and adherence to the regimen (see Chapter 13). Intensive management can be safely and successfully applied to the care of a youth with diabetes only if the family has the requisite emotional and economic resources. The cost of intensive therapy is approximately twice that of conventional therapy. The ability and willingness of a family to assume any additional expenses they must bear may be an important factor limiting the clinician's ability to intensify a patient's management.

The Adherence Problem

Adherence to a complex, demanding, intensive diabetes regimen requires lifelong changes in behavior and involves repeated daily performance of several unpleasant tasks: injections, SMBG, meal planning, and exercise routines. Only a minority of patients complies with all the elements necessary to achieve optimal glycemic control. Poor adherence to the prescribed regimen, therefore, is a major impediment to maintaining optimal health of individuals with diabetes. Recurrent diabetic ketoacidosis is usually caused by major deviations from recommended therapy and, most importantly, from missed insulin injections. It is important to recognize the prevalence of mismanagement and candidly and nonjudgmentally discuss these behaviors with patients and their families.

- Make concrete strategies for minimizing mismanagement a standard part of diabetes education for all patients and their families. Address the patient's goals and earn his or her trust by being willing to compromise. Recommend small changes and implement them at a rate that the patient can tolerate.
- Encourage parents to play an active role in their adolescent's diabetes care. This notion may run counter to the conventional wisdom of allowing adolescents to assume increasing responsibility for their own management, but research and clinical experience reveal that increased parental involvement and supervision are effective in decreasing nonadherence, preventing ketoacidosis, and improving glycemic control in teenagers.
- Sharing the burden of care with family members is especially important when the adolescent patient is not achieving the goals of therapy. Determine the appropriate degree of parental involvement by the adolescent's success in self-management.

CONCLUSION

Although improving diabetes control in adolescents is an arduous task for patients, families, and health care providers, the diabetes clinician cannot shrink from the challenge. Any sustained reduction in the level of glycated hemoglobin lowers the risk of diabetic microvascular and neuropathic complications. Therefore, clinicians should use all the resources at their disposal and make a concerted effort to help the adolescent patient with diabetes to prevent deterioration of glycemic control during the adolescent years and to achieve near-normal glycemia.

BIBLIOGRAPHY

American Diabetes Association: Standards of medical care for patients with diabetes mellitus (Position Statement). *Diabetes Care* 24 (Suppl. 1):S33–S43, 2001

Amiel S, Sherwin R, Simonson D, Lauritano A, Tamborlane W: Impaired insulin action in puberty: a contributing factor to poor glycemic control in adolescents with diabetes. *N Engl J Med* 31:215–219, 1986

Anderson BJ, Ho J, Brackett J, Finkelstein D, Laffel L: Parental involvement in diabetes management tasks: relationships to blood glucose monitoring adherence and metabolic control in young adolescents with insulin-dependent diabetes mellitus. *J Pediatr* 130:257–265, 1997

Bojestig M, Arnqvist HJ, Hermansson G, Karlberg BE, Ludvigsson J: Declining incidence of nephropathy in insulin-dependent diabetes mellitus. *N Engl J Med* 330:15–18, 1994

Boland EA, Grey M, Oesterle A, Fredrickson L, Tamborlane WV: Continuous subcutaneous insulin infusion: a new way to lower risk of severe hypoglycemia, improve metabolic control, and enhance coping in adolescents with type 1 diabetes. *Diabetes Care* 22:1779–1784, 1999

Connell J, Thomas-Dobersen D: Nutritional management of children and adolescents with insulin-dependent diabetes mellitus: a review by the diabetes care and education dietetic practice group. *J Am Diet Assoc* 91:1556–1564, 1991

Delahanty L, Halford B: The role of diet behaviors in achieving glycemic control in intensively treated patients in the Diabetes Control and Complications Trial. *Diabetes Care* 16:1453–1458, 1993

Diabetes Control and Complications Trial Research Group: Effect of intensive diabetes treatment on the development and progression of long-term complications in adolescents with insulin-dependent diabetes mellitus: Diabetes Control and Complications Trial. *J Pediatr* 125:177–188, 1994

Krolewski A, Laffel L, Krolewski M, Quinn M, Warram J: Glycosylated hemoglobin and the risk of microalbuminuria in patients with insulin-dependent diabetes mellitus. *N Engl J Med* 332:1251–1255, 1995

Schmidt L, Colby P, Kwong C: Practical nutritional guidelines to reduce the risk of hypoglycemia in patients treated with insulin. *Clinical Diabetes* 13:46–48, 1995

Joseph I. Wolfsdorf, MB, BCh, is Director of the Diabetes Program and Chief of the Charles A. Janeway Medical Firm at Children's Hospital in Boston, MA. He is also an Associate Professor of Pediatrics at Harvard Medical School in Boston, MA.

15

Working with Young Adults Who Have Type 1 Diabetes

HOWARD A. WOLPERT, MD

Young adulthood is a transition period when lifelong routines of self-care are frequently set. In addition, this is a stage when complications from diabetes sometimes first manifest and when early intervention can be critical. Older teens tend to have a sense of "invulnerability" and underestimate the risks to their future health (see Chapter 13), and, unfortunately, many young adults with diabetes are lost to follow-up. Furthermore, the medical system, which is divided into separate pediatric and adult medicine tracks, has given relatively little attention to the special needs of this transitional age-group. There is often a misfit between the developmental tasks of the early young adult period and the responsibilities of diabetes self-management. Many clinicians expect the physically mature young adult to readily accept the demands of managing diabetes and give little consideration to the developmental context that affects the patient's self-care behavior. In this chapter, the developmental background to the young adult period will be reviewed, and several fundamental treatment principles will be outlined.

UNDERSTAND THE DEVELOPMENTAL PHASES OF YOUNG ADULTHOOD

The clinical and therapeutic approaches of the health care provider need to be framed in the context of the developmental stage of the young adult. In general, young adulthood comprises two overlapping developmental phases:

1. During the early phase (often corresponding to 18–22 years of age), relationships with parents change, and the individual moves from dependence to interdependence. Struggles with "authority" figures may continue, affecting how the health care professional engages with the patient. The overwhelming changes of this period (including graduating from high school, moving away from home, beginning new educational directions, and beginning to work and be self-supporting) may be a distraction from diabetes self-care, and the health care provider needs to consider these competing life priorities when setting up treatment goals with the patient.
2. During the late phase (often corresponding to 23–30 years of age), the focus of the individual shifts toward making choices and plans about future work directions, relationships, and lifestyle behaviors, and patients will often become receptive to improving their self-care. This period can present a window of opportunity for the health care provider to intervene and shape the habits that will determine the future health of the young adult.

RECOGNIZE CLINICAL PRINCIPLES

Develop a Collaborative Relationship

A key priority in caring for young adults with diabetes is developing a strong relationship that will ensure continued follow-up and that *over time* can be influential in promoting healthy self-care behavior. As pointed out by R. Anderson and Funnell in Chapter 1, the traditional model of medical care in which the health care provider prescribes the treatment plan does not conform with the practical realities of living with diabetes, where young adult patients must assume responsibility for their own care on a daily basis. As a counterpart to the new relationship that evolves between parent and child during the transition from adolescence to young adulthood, this phase of development should be accompanied by a reorientation of the provider-patient relationship to a collaborative model in which the provider serves as the patient's guide in making informed choices about living with diabetes. To underline that responsibility and control belong to the patient, it is often helpful for providers to explicitly describe themselves as the patient's "coach."

Assess the Developmental Stage and Receptiveness to Change of the Patient

The provider needs to sensitively assess the young adult's expectations and receptiveness to change and tailor the approach and treatment plans accordingly. The patient and provider will often have different perceptions of priorities in care. In contrast to patients presenting at a time of crisis (such as diabetes diagnosis or the onset of complications), when they usually expect the physician to be directive, asymptomatic young adults who are "graduating" from the pediatrician may not recognize the need for major changes in their diabetes regimen. Thus, unrealistic demands by the new physician with whom they have not yet developed a bond of confidence and trust may be perceived as an intrusion on their sense of personal control, and this can lead to estrangement from care and follow-up (see Chapter 2).

The challenges of the earlier phase of the young adult period will often be a distraction from the demands of managing the diabetes, and the patient will often not be receptive to major changes in the diabetes regimen. The focus of care may need to be directed at ensuring that the young adult has annual urine microalbumin measurements and dilated eye examinations, and counseling concerning issues such as contraception, the risks of hypoglycemia from binge drinking, coping with the impact diabetes has on relationships, and the challenge of integrating the demands of diabetes into a busy schedule. Establishing a relationship based on acceptance and mutual respect during this period can be critical when developing influence to later promote improvements in self-care habits. As patients mature and their focus shifts toward making choices and plans for the future, they will often become more receptive to changing their self-care behavior.

Recognize the Impact of Changing Family Roles and Relationships

The usually abrupt transfer to complete independence and responsibility for self-care that occurs when young adults with diabetes leave home can be unsettling for both them and their parents.

- The developmental maturity of the young adult is an important consideration in deciding when to transfer care from the pediatrician to the adult care provider. Some patients may find the overwhelming changes and demands of the early young adult years a distraction from forging ties with a new physician. The young adult who is facing a difficult adjustment to college and has strong bonds with the pediatric team may do better if the transfer to adult medicine is delayed until after the college years.
- The health care provider needs to be attuned to anxieties that parents may develop as their involvement recedes during their child's passage to independence. Anxious parents who are overly intrusive and controlling can trigger a destructive cycle of "miscarried helping" that undermines their child's self-confidence and motivation. Making the parents aware that their well-intentioned efforts are being counterproductive can help break this cycle (see Chapter 19). In addition, parents will need ongoing reassurance as they disengage from their child's care, and it is often important for the physician to maintain contact with them during this process.

The health care provider needs to be attuned to the interaction between diabetes and the developing social relationships of the young adult.

- Misunderstandings related to the behavioral changes that occur with unrecognized hypoglycemia are common and can disrupt relationships. Other issues such as unrealistic expectations and blame can sabotage relationships and undermine self-care. Inviting the participation of partners in medical visits can help uncover these problems.
- The period when the young adult patient starts to develop permanent relationships and plans for the future will often signal a stage of receptiveness to improving self-care. Life partners can become influential agents for change, and it is often important to engage them in discussions about treatment options and plans.

Build Motivation to Change Self-Care Behavior

The clinician's task in building motivation and overcoming ambivalence about change in self-care behavior is complex and sometimes daunting. There are several aspects to this process.

Reshape perspectives about intensive therapy

Simply telling patients about the benefits of intensive therapy is rarely effective in persuading them to change self-care behavior. To develop effective communication between provider and patient, there needs to be a convergence of perspectives and goals. The physician will often focus on setting up the treatment plan, i.e., telling patients what they need to do to improve diabetes control. In general, health care professionals emphasize the benefits of good glycemic control while undervaluing the personal costs. In contrast, when looking at the implications of therapy, patients are often more concerned about the immediate costs, demands, and sacrifices and tend to lose sight of future benefits.

These contrasting perspectives highlight two important considerations:

1. The focus in care should not be directed exclusively at improving glycemic control but should be framed in terms of *making the diabetes more manageable.*
2. When introducing the patient to the tools of intensive diabetes management, the message of the provider needs to be reoriented to the patient's perspective, i.e., the message should include the more immediate and direct benefits of multiple injections and pump therapy in providing a *flexible, individualized* treatment program that fits into the demands of life.

Focus on the more immediate benefits

⇓

Overcome ambivalence about change

⇓

Promote engagement in self-care

⇓

Improve in glycemic control

Uncover barriers

Helping patients to identify personal hurdles can be a critical element in the path to better diabetes control:

- Misconceptions that equate intensive diabetes control with intensive self-control are unfortunately too common. Explaining to the patient that every 1% decline in glycated hemoglobin A1C (A1C) is equivalent to reducing his or her mean blood glucose level by 20–22 mg% will often help the patient to appreciate that intensive glycemic control is within reach.
- Exploring the patient's formative experiences with diabetes professionals may uncover a legacy of unrealistic perfectionist strivings that can set the patient up for frustration and disengagement (see Chapter 21).
- A history of severe hypoglycemic reactions should prompt exploration of whether fear of hypoglycemia underlies the patient's reluctance to intensify therapy.
- Concerns about weight gain associated with intensification of glycemic control are particularly common in the young adult population and need to be discussed openly and respectfully. Use of insulin pumps and glargine insulin can eliminate the need for extra unwanted snacking between meals and allows patients to more effectively exercise to burn off calories without the need for carbohydrate loading.

Set realistic goals

Goal setting has an important role in the complex process of behavioral change.

- Realistic, attainable goals that are appropriate for the patient's aptitude, motivation, and stage of development will reinforce the patient's sense of confidence and self-efficacy, and this can drive further progress as the goals are further advanced.
- Conversely, goals that are too ambitious and that overlook the realities of the patient's life (such as the competing priorities faced by a college student) and the complex difficulties of managing diabetes can set the patient up for failure, frustration, and disengagement from care.

Because improved self-care practices underlie improved A1C and blood glucose levels, goal setting should focus on self-care behavior in addition to biological targets. Goals need to be set in collaboration with the patient, and the patient must be able to relate to the goal at a practical level. For example, patients who are athletic will relate to the importance of optimizing glycemic control around exercise, and this can be a starting point for engaging them in improving their self-care. Supper will usually vary from day to day, and patients will often relate to the value of adjusting the suppertime insulin dose ("just as your pancreas would if you didn't have diabetes") to cover variations in food intake. This scenario can be used to introduce the patient to the concepts of carbohydrate counting and physiological insulin replacement. New self-care habits need to become an integrated part of daily routines, and, to ensure that the patient does not feel overburdened, changes in the diabetes regimen will often need to be introduced gradually.

Having realistic expectations and goals minimizes the risk for frustration and "diabetes burnout." During some of the transitions of the young adult period (such as leaving home, starting college, or starting a new job), even some of the more conscientious patients will have difficulty giving diabetes a high priority. Patients and parents will often need to be reminded that this is usually a normal transitory phase and not a sign of personal failure.

Minimize performance pressure about glycemic control

Because hyperglycemia is such an important factor in the development of the microvascular complications of diabetes, glucose control has become the measure of success in managing diabetes. Blood glucose monitoring is a crucial tool in the management of diabetes, and patient glucose records are now a major focus of the patient-provider interaction in diabetes. However, for the individual patient, blood glucose and A1C levels are more than just objective measures of glycemic control, but translate into a complex judgement of performance, competence, and self-worth. Minimizing this "performance pressure" can be a key element in reducing "burnout" and keeping the patient focused on monitoring glucose levels and optimizing diabetes control.

The health care provider can minimize performance pressure by:

- Helping the patient to appreciate that blood glucose monitoring is a tool ("compass") to direct diabetes management rather than a performance measure ("test").

- Individualizing blood glucose and A1C targets rather than focusing on an "ideal" and often unattainable "standard."
- Describing glucose and A1C levels with neutral language rather than judgmental expressions (for example, "high" instead of "poor" or "bad").

Recognize Your Impact on the Mental Health of the Patient

Health care providers have an important role in fostering the mental health of the patient with diabetes. Depression, lack of motivation, and disengagement from self-care can be the unintended consequence of the interactions between the patient and health care professional (see Chapter 3).

- **Reduce self-blame.** The Diabetes Control and Complications Trial and other intervention studies have established the causal link between glycemic control and the microvascular complications of diabetes. The positive message is that individuals with diabetes have some control over their destiny. However, patients will often perceive another message in this causal link: they are to blame for their complications. It is often overlooked that glycemic control is not the entire story: some individuals with relatively low A1C levels develop complications, and others with poorer control seem to be protected. Reminding the patient that "bad luck genes" predispose individuals to complications can help reduce the cycle of self-blame, despair, and lack of motivation that sometimes develops when complications strike.
- **Avoid "fear-mongering."** Many patients with diabetes live with a burden of fear and anxiety about complications and disability that is often unwittingly reinforced by health care professionals. Complications do not escape mention in educational materials on diabetes, and few patients need any reminder of the consequences of neglecting their self-care. There is no evidence that "fear-mongering" is successful in motivating patients. On the contrary, if the interaction with the health care professional heightens the patient's fears and anxieties, withdrawal from follow-up and self-care will often result (see Chapter 20).
- **Lessen the burden of fear.** Health care providers have an important role in reducing the burden of fear and anxiety that their

patients suffer. Although diabetes is the most common cause for blindness in the industrialized world, only a small fraction of individuals with diabetes develop severe visual loss. Patients should be aware that with timely use of laser therapy and surgery, <1% of individuals with proliferative retinopathy progress to legal blindness. Urine microalbumin testing allows for the detection of the earliest stage of diabetic nephropathy, and early intervention with angiotensin-converting enzyme inhibitors can substantially change the natural history of this complication.

CONCLUSION

The clinician will often have a rewarding opportunity to affect the future health of the young adult with diabetes. The treatment approach needs to be tailored according to the developmental stage, receptiveness, and expectations of the young adult. There are marked individual variations in the pace of maturational development, and, often, several years of relationship-building and collaboration between the provider and patient are required to effect change in self-care behavior. Patience and respectfulness toward the patient are the underpinnings to success in this process.

BIBLIOGRAPHY

Dunning PL: Young adult perspectives of insulin-dependent diabetes. *Diabetes Educ* 21:58–65, 1995

Wolpert HA, Anderson BJ: Managing diabetes: are doctors framing the benefits from the wrong perspective? *Brit Med J* 323:994–996, 2001

Wolpert HA, Anderson BJ: Young adults with diabetes: need for a new treatment paradigm. *Diabetes Care* 24:1513–1514, 2001

Wysocki T: Graduating to adult care. *Diabetes Self-Management* 11:41–43, 1994

Zhang L, Krzentowski G, Albert A, Lefebvre PJ: Risk of developing retinopathy in Diabetes Control and Complications Trial type 1 diabetic patients with good or poor control. *Diabetes Care* 24:1275–1279, 2001

Howard A. Wolpert, MD, is Senior Physician in the Section of Adult Diabetes at Joslin Diabetes Center in Boston, MA.

16

Identifying and Treating Youth at Risk for Type 2 Diabetes

DEBORAH YOUNG-HYMAN, PhD, CDE

Currently, one in five schoolchildren is overweight or obese. This statistic represents a doubling in the prevalence of children who are overweight in the past decade and contributes to a significant increase in the number of children and adolescents diagnosed with type 2 diabetes. Unless intervention to modify weight takes place, an epidemic of type 2 diabetes in the pediatric and adolescent population can be expected within the next 10–20 years. Minority children and those whose families have fewer financial resources and lower levels of education are at a greater risk for becoming overweight. Clinicians may also come into contact with children and adolescents who are at risk because they are treating a family member who is overweight or obese, has weight-related diabetes, or has other related medical conditions, or because parents are concerned about their child's overweight status. Regardless of the source, identification of a child at risk provides the opportunity to begin intervention.

KNOW HOW WEIGHT-RELATED DIABETES DEVELOPS

The development of type 2 diabetes depends on the coexistence of two related conditions: insulin resistance secondary to chronic hyperinsulinemia and impairment of β-cell function. Children and adolescents undergo the same process of metabolic deterioration associated with being overweight that has been documented in adults. This process has been documented in overweight children as young as 5 years of age.

IDENTIFY CHILDREN AT RISK

The following are the various factors known to be associated with an increased risk for the development of type 2 diabetes in children and adolescents:

- family history of type 2 diabetes and obesity
- minority status, particularly for girls
- lower socioeconomic status
- overweight (greater than the 95th percentile for age- and sex-adjusted height/weight ratio—BMI)
- hyperlipidemia or hypertension (using the Joint National Committee on Prevention, Detection, Evaluation and Treatment of High Blood Pressure pediatric and National Cholesterol Education Program normative values)
- high percent total body fat relative to weight
- insulin resistance as evidenced by acanthosis nigricans, polycystic ovarian syndrome (PCOS), and/or elevated fasting insulin and/or glucose
- sedentary lifestyle
- excessive caloric intake above that needed for usual growth and development

ASSESS LIFESTYLE FACTORS

In addition to assessing medical risk (height, weight, waist-to-hip ratio, acanthosis nigricans, PCOS, fasting insulin, and glucose and lipid levels), eating patterns and activity level should be assessed to determine the risk of developing type 2 diabetes. It is important to ask young people and their parents about relevant behaviors and attitudes, including:

- **Child's nutritional intake.** Nutritional intake can be assessed using a variety of methods (see Chapter 7). The first method is a food-frequency questionnaire, which asks the child/adolescent to indicate the frequency of various food choices over a specified period of time. A second method is a 24-h dietary recall. The child (with the parent) is asked to report everything consumed (including liquids) over the past 24 h, including portion sizes. The same assessment can be done in the form of a 3-day food diary. When assessing children and adolescents, corroborate the foods and amounts reported between parents and the child.

- **Family eating patterns.** How many times a week does the family eat meals together? Who in the family prepares the food?
- **Child's usual activity level.** How many hours a day does the young person spend in sedentary activity (watching television, using computers and electronic games)? How many hours does the child spend in structured and unstructured aerobic and strengthening activities (walking and other activities)?
- **Parental attitudes toward weight and eating.** Do parents think it is okay to be "big"? Do they think their child is "overweight"? Do they think their child is at risk for developing diabetes or other medical conditions because of his or her weight? Do parents think they can help the child lose weight and stay healthy?

EDUCATE YOUNG PEOPLE AND PARENTS ABOUT HEALTH RISKS

A child who is overweight is at increased risk for developing type 2 diabetes, even if no other risk factors exist. Education is a first step to reducing that risk. Parents need to know that once risk factors are elevated, they will remain so unless the lifestyle habits of the child and family change. Risk factor modification is predicated on a plan to establish healthy eating and exercise habits in the child and reduce BMI.

SUPPORT PREVENTION EFFORTS

Children are in the process of establishing patterns of food intake and exercise. The most effective way to reduce the risk of developing type 2 diabetes in childhood is primary prevention, which begins in the home and is supported by the health care community.

- Encourage parents to make opportunities available for children to enjoy healthy eating and usual childhood activities, thereby instilling a basic positive attitude toward healthful living.

■ Encourage parents to keep up their own health maintenance behaviors; children are more likely to eat vegetables and fruits and to exercise when they see their parents doing so.

INTERVENE TO REDUCE RISK

The goals of intervention and prevention methods are essentially the same: decrease excess caloric intake, increase activity, and promote weight loss. The goals of risk factor intervention are to enhance insulin sensitivity and to reduce hyperinsulinemia that contributes to the loss of β-cell function.

RECOGNIZE LIFESTYLE FACTORS THAT CONTRIBUTE TO OVERWEIGHT AND TYPE 2 DIABETES

A variety of lifestyle factors contribute to the number of individuals who are overweight or obese. Diets high in saturated and partially hydro-genated fats, low levels of physical activity, and sedentary lifestyle have converged in the past 20 years to produce an unprecedented epidemic of obesity and type 2 diabetes in adults and children. These lifestyle habits are facts of life for most busy American families. As of 1995, the average American eats food away from home for 27% of all eating occasions, with children consuming an average of 11% of daily energy consumption from fast food. Children watch television or engage in other sedentary activities 3–4 h per day (excluding school) and vigorously exercise, on average, <1 h each day. While watching television, children view literally hundreds of advertisements skillfully designed to increase the consumption of prepared and fast foods. The ready availability of fast foods discourages eating together in the home as a family, when parents can model and foster healthy eating habits. Finally, few adults are as active as they should be, and the environment where children spend more time than any other place—schools—have spent less time and devote fewer resources to ensuring physical activity and fitness at a time when such efforts are desperately needed.

These factors contribute to the risk of obesity and type 2 diabetes in all families, but especially families with limited financial resources—particularly those living in urban communities. These families generally find it harder to find and buy healthy foods, and it may be unsafe for children to be active outdoors. Cultural beliefs about body size combined with "optimistic bias" about children's vulnerability to disease may contribute to the lack of recognition of health risks related to weight and other risk factors.

Some suggestions for promoting healthy eating and exercise habits are:

- Make sure children have the opportunity for safe outdoor play by offering to be outside with them. Plan activity into every day, even if it is just a 20-min walk. Include the child's friends.
- Include children/teens in menu planning and trips to the grocery store. Teach kids cooking skills for healthy food choices. Reduce the amount of sweets and foods high in fat in the home. Substitute "healthy" snacks. Suggest that *everyone* in the home eat the same healthy food.
- Help parents to *not* reward their children with food for good deeds. Teach parents to offer praise, shared time, and activities for accomplishments. Reward and praise kids for physical activity. Do not punish a child by withholding an opportunity to exercise (see Chapter 8).

FACILITATE PARENT EMPOWERMENT

Many parents do not recognize the inherent health risks to overweight children. Help parents see when baby fat becomes overweight and what a healthy weight is for their child or adolescent. Show parents growth charts to see how their child's weight and height compare with those of other children the same age. This information can help parents and children recognize the range of normal heights and weights and where the child falls within that range. Parents whose primary culture is accepting of large body size may need education regarding the fact that overweight status in children as well as in adults is a health risk.

Parents need help making lifestyle changes and helping their children do the same. Parents may bristle or feel guilty if they perceive health care providers are implying that they lead a lifestyle harmful to their child. Parents may also need assistance in educating other family members or their community about the importance of lifestyle changes to prevent diabetes.

When children are weighed and measured during their usual health care visit, providers can talk about risk factors and prevention behavior, including ways to promote health without disrupting the social and family environment. Put aside time during visits to discuss how parents will incorporate healthful behaviors into their lives and their children's lives. There is no formula for reducing health risks. Each child and family will come to their own balance of habits and activities. Listen to what the child and family say they are willing to do to change behavior. The provider, the child, and the family should agree on goals.

Promoting healthful behavior can become an empowering experience for parents, but only if barriers to adopting a healthier lifestyle are discussed and addressed. Table 16.1 lists barriers that parents express and some suggested strategies for overcoming each barrier.

Tips for Parents

1. Model healthy eating in the home, with *all* family members eating the same foods. Have healthy "kid food" choices readily available, especially for snacks.

2. Exercise regularly. Be a role model for your child. If you are active and enjoy it, your child is more likely to be active as well. Ask your child to join you in physical activity, like a bike ride after dinner, instead of settling down in front of the television. Make sure exercise is fun, not just an obligation.

3. Reward and praise children and adolescents for being active every day. Enroll children in school- and community-sponsored sports activities. Attend the practices and games. Advocate school- and church-based activity programs. Offer to be the coach.

4. Talk with children about health risks. Let them know how they can improve their health. Advocate diabetes and heart disease prevention in your child's health curriculum and healthy choices on the school menu.

5. Make healthy eating choices taste good. Cook and eat meals together to monitor your child's nutrition intake and activities.

6. Read nutrition labels on packaged foods. Choose foods that are lower in fats and simple carbohydrates.

7. Discourage eating while watching television or while engaged in other sedentary activities. Inattention to food intake makes it hard to recognize feelings of fullness and can lead to overeating.

TABLE 16.1 **Strategies for Overcoming Barriers to Adopting a Healthier Lifestyle**

Barriers	Strategies
Lack of resources. Lack of money, poor health. Being a single parent stops me from cooking, exercising, watching my children, etc.	Identify people with whom to share child-care tasks who will help you monitor food intake and activity. Identify community resources to address financial and insurance needs.
Lack of opportunities for exercise. No safe place to play in neighborhood. School doesn't have a safe place to play outside or have regular physical education classes.	Advocate for increased opportunities. Find out if YMCAs and YWCAs have sliding scales or reduced fees for children. Enter the child in a sports league. Coach your child's team.
Fatalistic attitudes. What can I do about it? We are all big. I have never been able to do anything about my weight. Diabetes runs in our family.	Offer referral to a diabetes education program.
Lack of knowledge/cultural bias. This is the way we have always done it in my family. Other family members aren't fat; why should I make them change the way they eat?	Refer to a dietitian. Suggest participation in a community-based culturally specific weight management group for parents and children. (Weight Watchers, hospital, community center– or church-sponsored weight loss programs)
Lack of confidence in helping child change behavior. I don't know how to change my child's eating habits. I don't want to make my child unhappy. He won't listen to me. She just wants to be like her friends. I've given up. It's too much of a fight.	Teach monitoring of nutrition intake and activity and use of incentives for compliance with recommendations (e.g., use a chart to record goals and rewards). Refer to an individual, family support, or therapy group, or commercial weight management program. Suggest parent skills training, counseling, or group support to help empower parents as agents of change (Systematic Training for Effective Parenting [STEP] and Parent Effectiveness Training [PET] programs)

INCLUDE THE YOUNG PERSON

Children need to be actively involved in the process of healthy food and activity choices as soon as they are able, depending on the developmental stage of the child. Young children wish to please parents and will adopt behaviors (including nutrition choices) that are modeled and praised by parents (see Chapter 12). Middle-school children still hold to family values about food and exercise, although they may take some liberties when with friends. Teens are more influenced by peers; therefore, peer-based, structured, monitored, health-promoting activities are recommended to facilitate change in nutrition and exercise patterns. These activities are most likely to succeed if they are embedded in the teen's usual environment and are attended with friends. School, church, and youth-focused groups that promote healthy living activities without the label of "education" or "therapy" are more acceptable to teens.

Church-based youth groups often offer regular opportunities for physical activity, such as Habitat for Humanity projects and youth basketball/volleyball leagues for boys and girls. Peer-based weight management support groups that meet at a school have also been found to be acceptable to teens. Teens in particular need to express motivation to lose weight and often need "structure" imposed by having a diet plan, partner with whom to exercise, etc. It is important to avoid making healthy eating and activity "control" issues between parents and teens (see Chapter 13).

CONCLUSION

The key to preventing type 2 diabetes is identifying and treating risk factors. Preventing type 2 diabetes in children begins with the education of parents, health care providers, and the public: overweight status in children is not benign and brings health risks. Risk factors need to be assessed, monitored, and, if present, treated by engaging the family in health education coupled with a process of ongoing lifestyle modification. It is particularly important that interventions to modify risk factors begin immediately and be continued on a long-term basis.

BIBLIOGRAPHY

American Diabetes Association: *Medical Management of Type 2 Diabetes.* 4th ed. Alexandria, VA, American Diabetes Association, 1998

American Diabetes Association: Type 2 diabetes in children and adolescents (Consensus Statement). *Diabetes Care* 23:381–389, 2000

Anderson RE, Funnell MM, Fitzgerald JT, Marrero DG: The diabetes empowerment scale. *Diabetes Care* 23:739–743, 2000

Caprio S, Tamborlane W: Metabolic impact of obesity in childhood. *Pediatric Endocrinology* 28:731–747, 1999

Centers for Disease Control and Prevention: Update: prevalence of overweight and obesity among children, adolescents and adults: United States: prevalence trends, 1988–1994. *MMWR Morb Mortal Wkly Rep* 46:198–202, 1997

Falkner B, Michel S: Obesity and other risk factors in children. *Ethn Dis* 9:284–289, 1999

Haffner SM, Miettinen H: Insulin resistance: implications for type II diabetes mellitus and coronary heart disease. *Am J Med* 103: 152–162, 1997

Lin B-H, Guthrie J, Frazão E: Nutrient Contribution of Food Away from Home. AIB-750, Economic Research Service, U.S. Department of Agriculture, 1999

Young-Hyman D, Schlundt DG, Herman L, De Luca F, Counts D: Evaluation of the insulin resistance syndrome in 5- to 10-year-old African-American children. *Diabetes Care* 24:1359–1364, 2001

Young-Hyman D, Schlundt D, Herman L, Scott D: Perception of health risk in parents of obese African-American children. *Obes Res* 8:241–248, 2000

Deborah Young-Hyman, PhD, CDE, is Scientific Review Administrator at the Center for Scientific Review at the National Institutes of Health in Bethesda, MD.

17

Preventing Type 2 Diabetes in Adults

ELIZABETH A. WALKER, DNSc, RN, CDE

The results of the recently completed Diabetes Prevention Program (DPP) tell us that type 2 diabetes can be prevented or delayed in the U.S. multi-ethnic population. Given the epidemic of type 2 diabetes in the U.S. and throughout the world, this is tremendous news. Can we now assume that the type 2 diabetes epidemic has just been stopped in its tracks? Unfortunately, that is probably not the case. Just because a preventive therapy is known and available does not mean that at-risk individuals will be identified or that they will adopt preventive therapies or behaviors.

Prevention of disease and treatment of disease can be two different sets of activities and mindsets. Even after diagnosis, the facts that diabetes is a *chronic* disease and that type 2 diabetes usually has a rather insidious onset add to the complexity of prioritizing and motivating health behaviors. The challenge for clinicians is to be aware of at-risk groups (e.g., overweight, ethnic minority groups) and to communicate to groups or individuals in their clinical practices that the risk of developing diabetes is present, but there *are* effective preventive treatments.

This chapter provides some practical suggestions, grounded in behavioral models, for promoting health care provider and patient assessment of the risk for type 2 diabetes and for improving communication about managing that risk. Current treatments for preventing or delaying the onset of diabetes are explored, along with the risks and benefits of these options.

HELP PATIENTS ASSESS THE RISK OF DEVELOPING DIABETES

Risk factors for developing type 2 diabetes, as learned from epidemiological studies, include impaired fasting glucose, overweight, sedentary lifestyle, family history of type 2 diabetes, a woman having had a baby weighing >9 lb at birth, and hypertension, among others. And certain ethnic minority groups, such as Hispanic, African American, Asian American, and American Indian have a greater prevalence of this disease (see Chapter 4). Armed with this information, health care providers should be able to identify groups and individuals in their practices who may be at increased risk for developing diabetes and in need of greater awareness of preventive strategies.

There are several means of assessing type 2 diabetes risk or identifying undiagnosed diabetes. In a community setting, the paper and pencil Diabetes Risk Test on the American Diabetes Association website (www.diabetes.org) is helpful in indicating who might benefit from a blood test to further screen for diabetes. Once in a health care facility or provider's office, the high-risk person may have either the more standard fasting plasma glucose test or an oral glucose tolerance test to assess for diabetes. If the tests are negative, preventive actions become key opportunities for both provider and patient.

The provider should consider initiating a discussion with any patient whose risk for developing diabetes is high. The patient's personal style (see Chapter 2) and prior experience with diabetes should guide the discussion. For example, if the individual assisted with a family member's diabetes care, especially if that family member had serious problems, such as a foot amputation or blindness, the discussion would cover very different emotional ground than a discussion with a person who has had no experience with diabetes. Risk reduction discussions will differ even among patients who have extensive experience with diabetes. One person may have a strong resolve to do everything possible to fight diabetes, while another may feel fatalistic and helpless about the possibility of preventing diabetes and its complications. Eliciting patients' personal experience of diabetes, their emotional response to this disease, and their beliefs about prevention can help them in acknowledging a personal risk of developing diabetes. Even though there are widespread public health messages about the risks of developing type 2 diabetes and diabetes complications, preventive actions are usually adopted when a person perceives his or her own personal risk.

RECOGNIZE HOW PATIENTS MAKE RISK REDUCTION DECISIONS

The protection motivation theory, developed by R.W. Rogers several decades ago, is a useful model to help clinicians understand how their patients make decisions about adopting healthy behaviors. Alternately, it may also help explain why patients may *not* adopt a provider's suggestions for behavior change. This model (illustrated in simplified form in Figure 17.1) portrays some of the cognitive processes of interest when a person is considering behavioral changes for self-protection (e.g., to prevent type 2 diabetes). The following example can be traced from left to right in Figure 17.1. A woman considers the *rewards* of an unhealthy behavior (e.g., frequent lunches of cheeseburgers and fries) in relation to the *severity* of the threat, such as developing type 2 diabetes, and the probability that the threat may happen to her (i.e., her *vulnerability*). *Fear,* as an emotional response, may have an indirect influence on her appraisal of the threat's severity. This emotional factor helps to explain why past experience with diabetes is an important piece of information for the clinician. Sometimes emotions can "short circuit" information processing (see Chapter 20).

At the same time, the person may also be considering how effective she believes eating healthier lunches might be to help prevent diabetes (i.e., *treatment efficacy*) and whether she can really make and sustain that change (her *self-efficacy* to modify her lunch menu). The *costs* are what she believes she must give up (her comfort foods) to adopt this new behavior of choosing healthier foods at lunch. When the balance of the *threat appraisal* and the *coping appraisal* tips in favor of adaptive coping (eating healthier lunches to help prevent diabetes), her motivation to *act* to protect herself is bolstered. The patient's mental process of appraising threats and coping skills may occur in a matter of seconds during or after a clinical encounter. An important issue for clinicians is to broaden their understanding of factors contributing to what may *appear* as their patient's complacency or denial in the face of a health risk, such as the risk of developing diabetes. Appreciating the thought processes in the

Cognitive Mediating Process

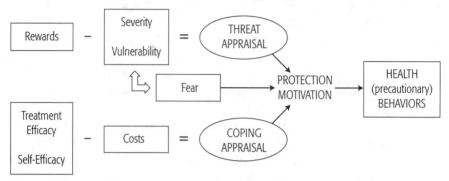

FIGURE 17.1 A simplified version of the model for protection motivation theory. Adapted from Rogers RW, Prentice-Dunn S: Protection motivation theory. In *Handbook of Health Behavior Research I: Personal and Social Determinants.* Gochman DS, Ed. New York, Plenum Press, 1997, p. 113–132.

model (Figure 17.1) should enhance the discussion of both risk and preventive behaviors when the appropriate opportunity arises between patient and provider.

CURRENT OPTIONS FOR PREVENTING OR DELAYING TYPE 2 DIABETES

Several recent studies, including the DPP, have shown that type 2 diabetes can be prevented or delayed. The Finnish Diabetes Prevention Study showed that middle-aged Finnish subjects with impaired glucose tolerance could implement a lifestyle modification intervention (diet and physical activity) and lower their risk of developing diabetes by 58% when compared with a control group. An earlier report from Da Qing, China, also showed promising results in diabetes prevention from lifestyle modification of diet and exercise. The DPP was undertaken in the U.S. to test hypotheses about prevention of type 2 diabetes in a multi-ethnic, high-risk population, with almost 20% of the sample over 60 years of age. Participants were randomized either to an intensive lifestyle intervention of diet and increased physical activity or to the antihyperglycemic agent, metformin, with its corresponding placebo. Results of the DPP were highly encouraging. Participants in the lifestyle intervention group developed diabetes during the course of the study at a rate 58% lower than participants in the placebo group. The benefits of the lifestyle intervention are particularly striking because the goals for participants in this study group—reducing body weight by 7% and being physically active 150 min/week—are within the reach of many people. Also impressive was the fact that the positive health benefits of the DPP lifestyle intervention applied to all age and ethnic groups and both sexes. As noted, the DPP medication intervention (850 mg metformin twice each day) reduced the rate of progression from impaired glucose tolerance to diabetes by 31% when compared with the placebo group; the medication was about half as effective as the lifestyle intervention and less effective in individuals with a lower BMI and in individuals ≥60 years of age.

The take-home message for clinicians is that there are definitely efficacious interventions to prevent type 2 diabetes in men and women of all ages and ethnic groups who are at high-risk for developing type 2 diabetes because they have impaired glucose tolerance. Increasing public awareness of these preventive strategies and providing effective means to implement them is paramount.

INCREASE THE CHANCES OF COMMUNICATING EFFECTIVELY

How can the provider have a prevention dialogue with a patient when there are other current health problems to discuss during the visit? Should the provider use statistics regarding risk, morbidity, mortality, and prevalence rates for groups? In the risk communication literature, the emphasis has turned away from statistics and numbers, which are often difficult to comprehend at a personal level. There is a movement toward stories and narratives about risks, so that people can relate this information to their life and experience. A sense of trust in the provider and the health care system is clearly important. The person's emotional response to the topic of diabetes prevention may make it either a priority for prompt attention or a topic easily disregarded.

What else is going on with the patient at the time of the prevention discussion? Comorbid issues, family problems, lack of social support, and acute health priorities are all competing demands on a person's attention. A model to help assess where to begin the prevention discussion is the psychologist N.D. Weinstein's precaution adoption process model (Figure 17.2). This model is similar to J. Prochaska's stages of change (transtheoretical) model, although elements of the precaution adoption process model are particularly pertinent to preventive actions. Figure 17.2 portrays the basic, intuitive process. At the left, the model starts with a person *unaware* that he may be at high risk for type 2 diabetes. He may think, "There's no diabetes in my family, so I won't get it." Another individual may be *aware* of his higher risk status (e.g., that he is middle-aged, Hispanic, and overweight), but he is *unengaged* by the idea of this risk. Perhaps he is focused on other acute health problems. But after speaking with his primary care provider, he decides that he should, at least, listen to the issues and therapeutic options for preventing type 2 diabetes. The gentleman will either *decide to act* to prevent diabetes, or *not to act*, over a period of time. If and when he decides to act to prevent diabetes, the actions he chooses will depend on many beliefs, including treatment efficacy ("How well will these pills work?") and his self-efficacy ("Am I able to change my diet and exercise more?") regarding treatment choices. Once the individual *takes action*, the critical issue is the *maintenance* preventive behavior. Will this behavior remain a priority in the face of competing demands on his energies?

Maintaining prevention behavior requires that the patient be prepared to manage potentially challenging situations. For example, a person who decides to eat healthier lunches must be prepared to deal with the temptations posed when coworkers suggest everyone go out to lunch at a fast-food restaurant. Their regular fare (a cheeseburger and fries) tastes good, and the social experience is enjoyable as well. In addition, when faced with this high-risk situation, the patient might not feel as confident that diabetes prevention is important or possible.

You may think that maintaining the behavior of "just taking a pill" to prevent diabetes would be easy for most people; however, there are many reasons why some people prefer not to take medications, especially when the therapeutic benefit is not clear and direct, such as taking an effective analgesic for acute pain. Helping patients take preventive medications on a regular basis is easier when the medication-taking behavior is incorporated into an established daily routine. For example, if a person always takes blood pressure pills or a daily vitamin, suggest that the diabetes prevention pill be stored with and taken at the same time.

Patients need to feel confident that *this time* it can work for them. The health care provider's role is to help the patient embark on a pre-

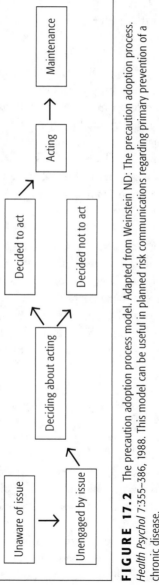

FIGURE 17.2 The precaution adoption process model. Adapted from Weinstein ND: The precaution adoption process. *Health Psychol* 7:355–386, 1988. This model can be useful in planned risk communications regarding primary prevention of a chronic disease.

ventive course of action such as lifestyle modification. Again, the key is helping patients keep in mind their motivation for prevention efforts and developing personal solutions to the daily challenges they face when maintaining these efforts.

Health behaviors may be preventive in nature, such as increasing physical activity, or they may be detection activities, such as getting screened for retinopathy. Studies of how to "frame" a health message use basic principles of decision science. The frame in this case is either *gain* (the benefits of adopting the behavior) or *loss* (the costs or risks from not adopting it). Research tells us that gain-framed messages (Table 17.1) are more effective in promoting prevention behavior. Alternately, loss-framed messages seem to promote detection behaviors more effectively.

The most effective gain-framed messages may be unique to the individual, and clinicians can help patients identify the messages they find most motivating. For example, a high-risk patient may express that he is highly motivated to prevent diabetes when he reminds himself that he wants to be alive to see his newborn grandson graduate from high school.

In contrast, a loss-framed message might be, "If you do not lose weight and increase your exercise, you are at high risk of getting diabetes and shortening your life." For prevention behaviors, this frame has been found to be less effective. Although loss-framed messages are appropriate for promoting certain behaviors such as screening for complications, diabetes prevention probably gains from a more positive spin to messages. For more on techniques to enhance self-care behaviors, see Chapter 1 on facilitating empowerment and Chapter 6 on fostering coping skills.

CONCLUSION

Type 2 diabetes can be prevented or delayed, but this does not ensure that high-risk individuals will adopt preventive treatments. The goal of this chapter was to give clinicians some practical strategies gleaned from behavioral science for communicating with appropriate patients about the risk of type 2 diabetes and current effective options for preventing this chronic disease.

The protection motivation theory is helpful for understanding what goes into a preventive decision—the weighing of the risks and benefits of taking action. The precaution adoption process model can assist the

TABLE 17.1 Gain-Framed Messages for Diabetes Prevention

- Losing weight and becoming more active increase your chances for enjoying a long, active, healthy life with your family.
- Taking this diabetes prevention pill as suggested can prevent or delay the onset of type 2 diabetes.
- Preventing diabetes is a gift of health for yourself and your family.

clinician in tailoring communications to greater benefit the patient by matching the message to the patient's stage of awareness and decision. Finally, gain-framed messages are usually more effective for fostering preventive health behaviors than loss-framed messages.

Adopting and maintaining preventive behaviors are major everyday challenges for most individuals. Clear, facilitative clinician-patient communication is the key to helping patients identify and resolve the myriad challenges to sustaining preventive behaviors.

ACKNOWLEDGMENTS

This work was supported in part by National Institutes of Health Grant DK-20541-24 and by the Rockefeller Foundation.

BIBLIOGRAPHY

Diabetes Prevention Program Research Group. Reduction in the incidence of type 2 diabetes with lifestyle intervention or metformin. *N Engl J Med* 346:393–403, 2002

Edwards A, Prior L: Communication about risk: dilemma for general practitioners. *Br J Gen Pract* 47:739–742, 1997

Fisher EB, Walker EA, Bostrom A, Fischhoff B, Haire-Joshu D, Johnson SB: Behavioral science research in the prevention of diabetes: status and opportunities. *Diabetes Care* 25:599–606, 2002

Pan XR, Li GW, Hu YH, Wang JX, Yang WY, An ZX: Effects of diet and exercise in preventing NIDDM in people with impaired glucose tolerance: the Da Qing IGT and Diabetes Study. *Diabetes Care* 20:537–544, 1997

Rogers RW, Prentice-Dunn S: Protection motivation theory. In *Handbook of Health Behavior Research I: Personal and Social Determinants.* Gochman DS, Ed. New York, Plenum Press, 1997, pp. 113–132

Rothman AJ, Salovey P: Shaping perceptions to motivate healthy behavior: the role of message framing. *Psychol Bull* 121:3–19, 1997

Slovic P: Perception of risk. *Science* 236:280–285, 1987

Tuomilehto J, Lindstrom J, Eriksson JG, Valle TT, Hamalainen H, Ilanne-Parikka P, et al.: Prevention of type 2 diabetes mellitus by changes in lifestyle among subjects with impaired glucose tolerance. *N Engl J Med* 344:1343–1350, 2001

Weinstein ND: The precaution adoption process. *Health Psychol* 7:355–386, 1988

Elizabeth A. Walker, DNSc, RN, CDE is an Associate Professor of Medicine and the Director of the Prevention and Control Component of The Diabetes Resaerch and Training Center at Albert Einstein College of Medicine in the Bronx, NY.

18

Caring for Elderly Patients with Diabetes

JOHN F. ZREBIEC, MSW, CDE

The number of people over 65 years of age in the United States continues to increase dramatically. By 2030, there will be 69 million older adults in the U.S., and individuals over 85 years of age will comprise the most rapidly growing segment of the population. Because the prevalence of diabetes is escalating, we can anticipate that cases of type 2 diabetes, the type of diabetes most common in the elderly, will proliferate among older Americans. In addition, the daily self-care demands of diabetes do not get any easier with age. Furthermore, nearly 20% of older adults experience mental disorders that are not part of normal aging, with the most common disorders including anxiety, depression, and cognitive impairment. In essence, the potential complications from diabetes, the frequent presence of comorbid chronic illnesses, and the social, functional, and psychological changes imposed by the aging process present older adults and their caregivers with special challenges. This chapter focuses on several psychological and behavioral strategies to help successfully care for the older patient.

UNDERSTAND THE NORMAL DEVELOPMENTAL TASKS OF AGING

Aging is a normal phase of life and not a pathological development. For most people, aging does not mean increasing depression or dementia, but these "golden years" are often not spent in carefree living, fishing, and baking cookies for the grandchildren. People are confronted with challenges to their intellectual vitality, social life, and sense of worth during the transition to retirement. The primary developmental tasks are to establish new roles and activities, tolerate the physical and cognitive changes of the aging process, accept the past, and discover a meaningful purpose for the remainder of life.

Certain life crises are a normal part of aging. Loss is the most important and difficult event, and grief is the most common emotional experience as a person loses spouse, family, and friends (see Chapter 20). Physical illness is the other major hurdle that faces the elderly. The ubiquitous preoccupation with the body and its functions is a normal consequence of aging, with the increasing probability of illness, hospitalization, surgery, pain, and disability. The possibility for developing complications from diabetes adds to this predictable challenge to remaining independent and productive.

For the clinician, it is important to consider the tasks that lie ahead for the patient, the capacity that is available to master those tasks, and the kind of help that is needed.

UNDERSTAND THE CLINICIAN'S PERSPECTIVE ON AGING

Clinicians' attitudes toward elderly patients affect the care that these patients receive. Difficulty in empathizing with older patients commonly occurs because the clinician:

- views diabetes as simply part of the aging process and, therefore, not very serious
- believes that elderly people cannot change or are too old to want to change, therefore making suggestions useless
- tends to infantilize the older person because he or she seems weak or vulnerable
- lets the patient's fears stimulate his or her own fears of old age, death, or the future
- lets the patient's conflicts trigger thoughts of his or her own personal conflicts

To avoid these problems:

- stay alert to inappropriate, exaggerated, ambivalent, erratic, or tenacious feelings toward the patient

- have a personal support system for discussion of feelings
- share care responsibilities with the rest of the team
- maintain an appropriate professional distance

UNDERSTAND THE PATIENT'S PERSPECTIVE ON AGING

Whereas elderly people are more likely to accept diabetes as part of the aging process, they are also more likely to perceive diabetes as less serious and, therefore, in less need of careful management. In addition, many older adults have other chronic illnesses that cause more suffering and require more attention. Basically, a person's perception about diabetes is an important factor in determining adherence. These perceptions often include beliefs about cause, seriousness, consequences, sense of control, and treatment effectiveness. One recent study found that beliefs about the effectiveness of treatment and the degree of satisfaction with medical care were the factors most predictive of dietary intake and physical activity. These beliefs about treatment, in themselves, result from a mixture of family attitudes about diabetes, past experiences with medical care, subjective distress due to complications or blood glucose results, and self-esteem.

The key point is that older people want to have their medical concerns listened to and taken seriously. It is imperative to ask patients about how diabetes affects their lives and what parts of diabetes care are difficult (see Chapter 1).

UNDERSTAND THE ROLE OF FUNCTIONAL STATUS

It is important to understand the elderly patient's functional status, that is, how the patient functions in activities of everyday living, such as fastening buttons or walking stairs. In fact, the patient's functional skills may be of more immediate importance than his or her metabolic status. Functional assessment is also crucial because practical medical management and realistic treatment goals rest upon an understanding of the capabilities of the older patient. A medical history may be helpful, but observation is key. For example, impaired hearing and vision can interfere with effective communication and the ability to understand educational directions or medical recommendations. Techniques such as eliminating extraneous noises, speaking slowly and in deep tones while facing the patient, writing questions in large print, and providing adequate lighting can be helpful. It is important to notice whether the patient:

- can see well enough to measure insulin, do blood glucose monitoring, and inspect his or her feet
- can hear well enough to understand medical recommendations
- is physically fit enough to climb stairs, handle a wheelchair, get on the examining table, get out of bed, open pill bottles, shop, cook, bathe and dress, or comply with exercise prescriptions to walk, swim, or bicycle
- is alert and oriented enough to remember medication regimens, dietary restrictions, and follow-up appointments

It is important to ask specific questions about symptoms and diabetes management because elderly patients tend to underreport details if they:

- are ashamed, misguided, or uneducated about diabetes
- expect illness as a normal part of aging
- fear illness
- want to please the clinician

For example, without detailed questioning, older people might never mention problems with sexual function because they are embarrassed, assume it is a consequence of aging, or are unaware of the effects of neuropathy.

Elderly patients with multiple complaints can frustrate the clinician who is trying to figure out the causes. These complaints, however, can be deceiving. Somatic complaints may be representations of underlying emotional distress in addition to symptoms of illness. Similarly, reports of physical illness may be exaggerated by emotional distress. In sorting out these complex dynamics, there is no substitute for spending time getting to know the patient. Yet, it is often not realistic to gather all the essential information in one long appointment that exhausts both the patient and the clinician. Shorter appointments with briefer agendas, spread over a few sessions, may prove more effective in gathering information without pressuring the older person.

IDENTIFY BARRIERS TO SELF-CARE

The lack of basic economic resources can have a tremendous impact on the older person. It can mean that the medical attention and supplies needed for diabetes care become secondary to the need for food, cloth-ing, and shelter. For example, adequate nutrition may be more impor-tant than blood glucose monitoring. The clinician needs to carefully assess income, housing, home care, resources (for food, clothing, trans-portation, utilities, personal care, and recreation), medical insurance, legal factors, and, of course, family support of patients. The clinician may need to be an advocate for the older person by not only taking responsibility for assessing the resources available, but also actually con-necting the patient with formal services. For example, a patient neither filled her prescriptions for metformin nor kept all her medical appoint-ments because she did not have a telephone or transportation. The doc-tor called in her prescriptions to the pharmacy and arranged for delivery, while a social worker arranged for free transportation to clinic appoint-ments. These strategies do require frequent, time-consuming health provider involvement with the patient, but the payoff in adherence to treatment recommendations is worth the effort.

SET SMALL, REALISTIC GOALS

Patients are likely aware of the unpredictable variations in daily routine that cause blood glucose problems. This awareness often makes them feel guilty and ashamed, and it does not help to blame patients or expect them to have more self-discipline. They have already had a lifetime in which to change habits, and it may now be a formidable task to ask someone to change a lifetime of eating and drinking in a certain way. It has been well documented that adherence to diabetes management is negatively influenced by the duration and extent of behavioral changes required and the complexity of treatment regimens. Few things will undermine motivation and create discouragement quicker than the inability to achieve a goal. Try to appreciate how small interventions can make a major impact on the quality of life.

Help patients make one or two changes at a time (see Chapter 6). For example, changing one item at breakfast may be a more realistic goal than revamping the person's entire meal plan. Easy armchair aerobics or walking may be more practical than going to a gym.

Many older people are afraid of the change from pills to insulin. Introducing the change through small steps may help alleviate their fears. For example, advise the patient to stay on oral agents while start-ing to take a small dose of intermediate-acting insulin at bedtime. This way, the patient gets used to handling syringes, finds that the injections are not like the immunizations remembered from youth, sees success and feels better, and is already on a split dose if he or she has to start morning insulin. Another technique is to ask the person to try insulin for 1 month to find out if he or she feels better.

INCLUDE THE FAMILY

A careful assessment of the elderly patient always requires a review of family and social support. Both research and clinical evidence suggest that family support has a positive impact on diabetes management. Often, family members are managers of the diabetes care, monitors of adherence with medical recommendations, and providers of transportation to appointments. Currently, nearly one of every four households in the U.S. provides care to a relative over 50 years of age. Most of these caregivers are women over 60 years of age, and studies have estimated that nearly 50% of these caregivers are overburdened and depressed.

Family meetings present an opportunity to evaluate caregiver burnout, openly discuss treatment plans, review realistic alternatives, and make treatment decisions that the family is able to understand and support. Family members often have a different perspective than the patient on day-to-day adherence to diabetes care. A comparison between the patient's self-report and family observations can provide valuable insight into the degree of social support and level of diabetes self-management. Eliciting this kind of information can then lead to a discussion about how to offer more help or different kinds of assistance (see Chapter 19).

STAY ALERT FOR SIGNS OF DEPRESSION

Depression may be three times more prevalent in people with diabetes than in the general adult population, and depression in the elderly is probably underrecognized and undertreated (see Chapter 22). The rate of suicide is highest among older adults compared with any other age-group and twice the national average for those over age 85. Depression is often the direct result of escalating complications from diabetes, the demands of management, or the frustrations of erratic blood glucose control. Decreased adherence to treatment, decreased physical activity, and poor glycemic control are, in turn, often the result of depression.

Depression often increases alcohol use, which is an important consideration when working with the elderly because of its psychological and physical side effects. Alcohol abuse is four times more common in older men than in older women. The clinician needs to ask whether the patient thinks (or others have mentioned) that alcohol consumption is a problem.

The diagnosis of depression is not easy. Some drugs, such as blood pressure and heart medications and tranquilizers, can cause depression. Moreover, the symptoms produced by hyperglycemia are often mistaken for depression. The diagnosis gets even more complicated when there is cognitive impairment. The distinction between depression and dementia is crucial because depression is reversible and often quickly responds to supportive treatment and antidepressant medications.

CONCLUSION

Understanding the psychosocial realities faced by the older person with diabetes is important when designing successful diabetes treatment regimens. This chapter has suggested several strategies for optimizing diabetes management in the elderly patient. Key components of these strategies are the inclusion of the patient's family in both functional assessment and diabetes treatment, and setting practical achievable goals. The underpinnings of this approach rely on the clinician's understanding of the normal developmental tasks confronting the older person, the psychological and functional challenges superimposed by diabetes, and a nonjudgmental attitude about aging and diabetes control.

BIBLIOGRAPHY

American Association for Geriatric Psychiatry: Geriatrics and mental health: the facts. Available at www.aagpgpa.org/prof/facts_mh.asp

Funnell MM, Merritt JH: The challenge of diabetes and older adults. *Nurs Clin North Am* 28:45–60, 1993

Miller KE, Zylstra RG, Standridge JB: The geriatric patient: a systematic approach to maintaining health. *Am Fam Physician* 61: 1089–1104, 2000

Mooradian AD, McLaughlin S, Boyer CC, Winter J: Diabetes care for older adults. *Diabetes Spectrum* 12:70–77, 1999

Saunders JT, Pastors JG (Eds.): Professional issues in facilitating lifestyle change for people with type 2 diabetes. *Diabetes Spectrum* 12:17–38, 1999

Wing RR, Goldstein MG, Acton KJ, Birch LL, Jakicic JM, Sallis JF Jr, et al.: Behavioral science research in diabetes: lifestyle changes related to obesity, eating behavior, and physical activity. *Diabetes Care* 24:117–123, 2001

John F. Zrebiec, MSW, CDE, is a Lecturer in Psychiatry at Harvard Medical School and Associate Director of Mental Health Services at Joslin Diabetes Center in Boston, MA.

19

Involving Family Members in Diabetes Treatment

BARBARA J. ANDERSON, PhD

Research has taught us that family support is a critical component of successful diabetes management for children, adolescents, and adults. For clinicians faced with caring for more and more patients in less and less time, extending diabetes care to include family members may seem unrealistic. But research indicates that family members can actually make the clinician's job easier and help the patient achieve optimum health and quality of life.

Forging an effective therapeutic alliance with patients' families does take time and effort (see Chapter 3). Family members do not automatically give the support that patients need. Support must be individually defined for each patient within each family system. Moreover, support is dynamic and changes over time, as the patient and family grow and change.

When the clinician begins to involve family members in diabetes treatment, two general guidelines are important. First, the patient must feel comfortable including family members in educational sessions. The clinician must make the boundaries clear—that his or her first responsibility and relationship is with the patient. All discussions about diabetes will take place with the patient present. Second, in families with severely dysfunctional interaction patterns or families in whom a member has serious psychiatric problems, successful involvement of the family in diabetes treatment may not be feasible.

In this chapter, the following five fundamental principles for successfully involving family members in diabetes treatment will be identified; then each will be discussed in detail.

1. Understand the impact of the patient's and family's cultural and/or religious practices on diabetes management (see Chapter 4).
2. Teach the family about diabetes and its treatment, beginning at diagnosis.
3. Listen to and identify diabetes-related feelings of family members. The family's concerns and worries about diabetes need to be addressed, and the family needs to learn that diabetes often brings a full range of feelings (e.g., fear, frustration, guilt, anger, etc.) (see Chapter 4).
4. Teach family members to have realistic and appropriate expectations concerning the patient's medical and behavioral goals.
5. Teach family members how to provide effective support without pushing or controlling the patient, which only serves to undermine the patient's own attempts at healthy diabetes self-care.

PRINCIPLES

Understand the Impact of the Patient's and Family's Cultural and/or Religious Practices on Diabetes Management

Because diabetes affects every facet of family life, the family's ethnic and religious heritage must be taken into consideration. The clinician needs to assess cultural and/or religious practices and beliefs that may affect management, such as calling for periods of fasting. The clinician should make every effort to be sensitive to and respectful of the patient's and family's views (see Chapter 3).

When religious or cultural barriers to diabetes management are present, it may helpful to seek guidance from another health care professional (physician, nurse, social worker, or educator) from the same or a similar culture to help "translate" the patient's and family's perspective to the clinician and the importance of specific diabetes guidelines to the family.

Type 2 diabetes is increasing at an alarming rate among several racial/ethnic groups in the U.S., such as Native Americans, African

Americans, and Hispanic Americans. All diabetes health care providers should seek diabetes education materials that are culturally sensitive. For example, the American Diabetes Association's *Diabetes Channel Series* is a patient-centered education series that is easy to read and has been developed and field-tested with diverse audiences.

Teach the Family About Diabetes and Its Treatment

At the time of diagnosis, encourage patients to bring in their family support person for an educational and getting-acquainted session, which can occur during a medical visit. The support person may be a spouse, a girlfriend or boyfriend, a roommate, a grandparent or sibling, or any other caregiver of the patient.

For established patients, invite them to bring in a supportive family member at any time. Many patients will not initiate a family meeting on their own. Some patients may state that they do not want help or support from anyone in their family. Encourage these patients to try to include and educate family members. However, if the patient continues to resist involving family members, this decision is the patient's right, and the clinician must respect this.

Use this session to begin general education about diabetes as a chronic disease with a complex medical treatment regimen. Tell family members about the possible causes of diabetes, changes in the treatment of diabetes over the past 20 years, and the impact of diabetes on many dimensions of family life—daily routines, finances, celebrations, and meal schedules.

Find out what the family believes or knows about diabetes. To learn about family beliefs about diabetes, ask a question such as, "How has diabetes affected people (family and friends) you know?"

Listen to and Identify Diabetes-Related Feelings of Family Members

Listening to the family's concerns about diabetes is not a recommendation to do family therapy, but rather family education. It is not critical to have a solution or answer for every feeling voiced by the patient's spouse or parent. What is important is that feelings are voiced and concerns are raised and that feelings based on mistaken beliefs are exposed as early in the course of the disease as possible. Diabetes normally brings into families a range of complex feelings, such as the following:

Guilt. Feelings of guilt are often a burden to parents or grandparents who believe that because diabetes is in their family, they are solely responsible for the diabetes. It is important to explain that no one gene causes diabetes and that no one side of the family is responsible for diabetes. State clearly that there are still many unanswered questions about the causes of diabetes but that current thinking is that diabetes comes from both sides of the family and is caused by environmental as well as genetic factors.

Blame. Blame can be crippling. It can prevent many patients from ever getting fully involved in their own diabetes self-care (see Chapter 20). In overweight patients with type 2 diabetes, it is a common mistake for family members to believe that overeating and excessive weight gain alone caused the diabetes. It is important to explain that scientists do not yet know all of the risk factors for type 1 or type 2 diabetes and are not yet able to prevent diabetes.

Financial concerns. Family members sometimes worry about the financial burden of diabetes supplies as well as about health and life insurance coverage for the patient. Diabetes does bring extra expenses into the family. Therefore, health insurance coverage is critical for people with diabetes. When concerns arise about financial and health insurance issues, they are often handled most effectively by referral to a skilled medical social worker. Local chapters of the American Diabetes Association and Juvenile Diabetes Foundation can sometimes help in finding the best buys in diabetes supplies at a local level.

Loss of a "normal lifestyle." Many family members worry that life will never again seem normal. Ask family members to identify their major concerns. Then begin to help the family address these concerns. Contact with a support group or with other families who have managed successfully may help to communicate that after a period of adjustment, most families achieve a *new* normal lifestyle.

Fears. Family members are frequently afraid of the long-term complications of diabetes. For these families, it is important to reassure them that all their efforts to help the patient maintain good blood glucose control are steps in helping to prevent long-term complications. In addition, point out that physicians can now identify signs of physical complications much earlier and that earlier detection and treatment may stop some complications from getting worse.

Discuss the many medical advances made over the past decades. Mention, for example, new oral medications, new types of insulin and schedules for insulin delivery, and new methods for monitoring blood glucose control, such as home blood glucose meters and the glycated hemoglobin A1C (A1C) test. When stable blood glucose control is maintained within the context of frequent medical follow-up, all of these new tools help to increase the patient's probability for a long and healthy life with diabetes. This may be a more optimistic message than many family members have heard before, and, therefore, it may need to be repeated and reinforced.

A second frequent fear of family members (which is much less discussed) is fear of low blood glucose. Seeing a loved one become incoherent or disoriented or have a seizure because of a low blood glucose reaction can be a terrifying experience for family members. Acknowledge this reality. Help family members understand that hypoglycemia is expected to occur in patients who are trying to improve their blood glucose control or are striving for tight control. Tell spouses that patients cannot always detect the warning signs of hypoglycemia but that some patients can learn to detect their early warning signs more accurately (see Chapter 11). Point out to family members that placing blame or indicating disappointment when the patient has a low blood glucose reaction only compounds the problem. Most importantly, teach family members to support the patient by readily stopping an activity so that the patient can check his or her blood glucose level or have a snack.

Family members need to understand what hypoglycemia feels like to the patient, and they need to realize that the patient may behave differently when experiencing it. Low blood glucose levels may cause moodiness or negative behavior in the patient or may make it unsafe, at times, for the patient to perform certain daily activities, such as driving, operating machinery, or caring for young children. Living with hypoglycemia and the threat of hypoglycemia are profound stresses on the family. Help families by anticipating and responding directly and realistically to the stress of hypoglycemia.

Family members can help patients in the prevention and treatment of hypoglycemia. Many family members feel helpless in the face of hypoglycemia. Therefore, it is important to tell them that by helping the patient prevent low blood glucose reactions, they are providing the most direct assistance possible. In some families, one person tries to see that the patient carries some fast-acting treatment for low blood glucose. Sometimes, a family member may carry a backup supply rather than ask or remind the patient. Some patients are helped when a family member reminds them to check their blood glucose. In other families, members learn to give glucagon just in case the patient has a severe low blood glucose reaction. Ask the patient and the family to decide what behaviors would work best for them.

To summarize this guideline about listening to the broad range of normal feelings—from fears of hypoglycemia to guilt over the diagnosis—that diabetes brings to all families, remember that while it is not necessary to supply answers for all of the family members' concerns, it is necessary and most useful to be informed about and sensitive to family members' concerns and to begin to try to address some of these concerns.

Teach Family Members to Have Realistic and Appropriate Expectations Concerning the Patient's Medical and Behavioral Goals

Teach family members that perfect blood glucose levels and perfect behavior are not possible goals in diabetes management. Similarly, help family members understand that patients with diabetes cannot always control their blood glucose levels, even if they are following their medical regimen. Without this foundation, family members assume that high and low blood glucose levels are always due to the patient's lack of behavioral control (e.g., "no will power," "lazy," etc.). When a family expects perfect blood glucose levels or diabetes management behavior from the patient, the patient is set up for failure and will experience more criticism and negative feedback from the family.

Help family members identify their unrealistic expectations for the patient's self-care behavior or for blood glucose levels or weight loss (see Chapter 6). Help family members see how having realistic expectations helps create more positive feelings between the patient and family members.

Teach Family Members How to Provide Effective Support Without Pushing or Controlling the Patient

Positive family involvement supports the patient's diabetes self-care. Destructive family involvement undermines the patient's attempts at healthy diabetes self-care. The process of learning to give support and help must be worked out for each family. Teach family members to ask the patient questions like, "Does it help you stay on your meal plan when I suggest that we go to the cafeteria instead of the snack bar for lunch?"

A "miscarried helping cycle" can occur when well-meaning efforts of family members leave patients feeling that family members lack confidence in them. Miscarried helping is when well-intentioned support attempts fail because they are excessive, untimely, or inappropriate. Second-guessing or arguing with the patient about his or her management decisions only undermines the patient's self-confidence and desire to make healthy choices. Even when family members know what to do, their helping effort may create a context that undermines the very objective they set out to achieve. Spouses and parents, especially, will feel frustrated that they cannot force the patient to make healthy choices all of the time. It is important to help families recognize that diabetes management at home will create conditions where the patient's motivation for self-care may become sidelined by the power of another struggle: that of preserving individual autonomy in the face of unwanted helping.

If a family is always arguing about "what is allowed on the meal plan," first ask patients to define what family members could do to help them stay on the meal plan. It may be that not eating treats in front of the patient would help most or that not eating all of the sugar-free ice cream out of the freezer would be a way family members could help. Helping may involve reminding or protecting the patient's special foods. Helping will be different with every patient and in every family. In miscarried helping, the original diabetes-related problem, such as the patient's need to adhere to a special meal plan, becomes lost or reframed. The helping process deteriorates when family members rely on strategies such as name-calling, insults, and other self-defeating behaviors. The patient feels shamed and blamed and increases his or her resistance. Everyone in the family has lost sight of the initial diabetes-related goal: the benefits to the patient of staying on a meal plan balanced with the medication.

In summary, it is not sufficient to simply tell family members they need to be helpful and supportive. Help define specific roles for each family member.

CONCLUSION

Family relationships play a vital, complex role in the lives of people with diabetes, and family support can have a positive effect on the metabolic control of the person with diabetes. For the clinician to begin to successfully involve family members in diabetes treatment, five principles are recommended:

1. Understand the impact of the patient's and family's cultural and/or religious practices on diabetes management.
2. Teach the family about diabetes and its treatment, beginning at diagnosis.
3. Listen to and identify diabetes-related feelings of family members.
4. Teach family members to have realistic and appropriate expectations concerning the patient's medical and behavioral goals.
5. Teach family members how to provide effective support without pushing or controlling the patient, which only serves to undermine the patient's own attempts at healthy diabetes self-care.

Providing diabetes information and support is often a delicate and highly individualized process for each patient and his or her family. The needs of both the patient and the family members must be addressed and balanced. Clinicians can assist families in negotiating this complex process by talking openly about the roles of family members.

ACKNOWLEDGMENTS

Preparation of this chapter was supported by the National Institute of Diabetes, Digestive, and Kidney Diseases Grant DKRO146887 and by the Charles Hood Foundation.

BIBLIOGRAPHY

Anderson BJ: Diabetes and adaptations in family systems. In *Neuropsychological and Behavioral Aspects of Insulin and NonInsulin Dependent Diabetes.* Holmes CS, Ed. New York, Springer Verlag, 1990, pp. 85–101

Anderson BJ: Working with families of patients on intensive insulin regimens. *Diabetes Spectrum* 8:69–70, 1995

Anderson BJ, Coyne JC: "Miscarried helping" in the families of children and adolescents with chronic diseases. In *Advances in Child Health Psychology.* Johnson J, Johnson S, Eds. Gainesville, FL, University of Florida Press, 1991, pp. 167–177

Baron RA: Negative effects of destructive criticism: impact on conflict, self-efficacy and task performance. *J Appl Psychol* 73:199–207, 1988

Butler D: For family members only. *Diabetes Self-Management* 19:7–10, 2002

Egede LE, Michel Y: Perceived difficulty of diabetes treatment in primary care: does it differ by patient ethnicity? *Diabetes Educ* 27:678–684, 2001

Gehling E: *The Family and Friends Guide to Diabetes: Everything You Need to Know.* New York, Wiley, 2000

Warram JH, Rich SS, Krolewski AS: Epidemiology and genetics of diabetes mellitus. In *Joslin's Diabetes Mellitus.* 13th ed. Kahn C, Weir G, Eds. Malvern, PA, Lea & Febiger, 1994, pp. 210–215

Barbara J. Anderson, PhD, is Research Investigator at Joslin Diabetes Center and an Associate Professor of Psychology at Harvard Medical School in Boston, MA.

Four

Understanding Psychological Issues That Affect Self-Care

Psychological well-being powerfully affects a person's capacity for diabetes self-management. In the first chapter of this part, Peyrot describes emotional responses to life with diabetes. He offers suggestions to help clinicians recognize and work with each of these responses.

Polonsky's chapter also addresses emotional responses to diabetes. This chapter describes how many people with diabetes feel overwhelmed and overstressed because diabetes care is never-ending, involves a variety of generally unpleasant tasks, and produces uncertain results, even when pursued aggressively. Polonsky focuses on practical strategies for preventing and treating diabetes burnout.

Depression in people with diabetes is a prevalent, chronic condition with consequences beyond the recognized effects of depression on emotional well-being. As Lustman, Singh, and Clouse point out, depression complicates diabetes management by influencing self-care, glycemic control, and the risk of long-term complications. The authors offer suggestions for treating depression in patients with diabetes, emphasizing the importance of effective depression treatment for improving mood, self-care, and glycemic control.

The desire to be thin is endemic among many adolescents and young women in our society. Recent research has shown that young women with diabetes are twice as likely to develop an eating disorder as young women without diabetes, in part due to the emphasis on diet and weight that is a fact of life for many people with diabetes. Studies show the destructive consequences of disordered eating for people with diabetes, including metabolic derangement and an increased risk for diabetes complications. In her chapter, Goebel-Fabbri explains how eating disorders develop and offers guidelines for detecting and treating eating disorders in young women with diabetes.

20

Recognizing Emotional Responses to Diabetes

MARK PEYROT, PhD

Emotions are an inherent part of the human response to stressful life situations, and diabetes involves several significant stressors. Major stress events include the onset and diagnosis of diabetes, changes in treatment regimen with the progression of the disease, and the onset and treatment of acute and chronic complications. Several stressful processes are involved in living with diabetes, including functional limitations, restrictions of lifestyle, threats to health, etc. It is important for clinicians to closely monitor emotional reactions to diabetes in their patients so that appropriate treatment can be instituted early, when the benefits are greatest. Effective treatment can restore emotional equilibrium—a worthy goal in its own right. Moreover, it is important for clinicians to address dysfunctional emotional responses because they may inhibit effective diabetes self-care. The goal of this chapter is to offer information and guidelines for treating emotional problems and disorders in individuals with diabetes.

BE AWARE THAT DENIAL AND FEAR ARE COMMON RESPONSES

Denial is a common response to diabetes, especially among patients with type 2 diabetes, because for them, diabetes onset is much less dramatic and the symptoms are often more subtle than those in patients with type 1 diabetes. Although most view denial as negative, this response is natural during a crisis; the negative consequences that may follow from denial, and not denial per se, are the problem. Denial can even be healthy if it protects patients from becoming emotionally overwhelmed. Maintaining emotional equilibrium is essential for establishing effective self-care.

Denial is maladaptive when it inhibits effective disease management, especially for extended periods. Maladaptive denial can be difficult to identify. The external appearance of not being concerned about diabetes and its management may result from two quite different foundations, only one of which is primarily emotional. On the one hand, patients may be unaware of the seriousness of diabetes. On the other hand, patients may be extremely threatened by diabetes and may use denial as a way of coping with their fear.

Another response to intense fear is catastrophizing or emphasizing the worst aspects of the disease, e.g., that you will get the complications of diabetes no matter what you do. This adaptation looks very different from denial, although it may have some of the same emotional antecedents and behavioral consequences. Patients who exhibit this response often feel overwhelmed and have given up as far as their self-care, i.e., they suffer from diabetes burnout. For more on working with patients who suffer from diabetes burnout, see Chapter 21.

Patients' fear-related responses can be ascertained indirectly by asking about diabetes-related attitudes and perceptions. Factors that may contribute to intense fear include perception of a need for unmanageable changes in lifestyle or a family history of diabetes-related poor outcomes. Lack of concern may result from a belief that diabetes has few consequences or from misinformation, such as the belief that if you do not have to take insulin, the diabetes is not serious.

Address Denial Directly and Effectively

Clinicians should avoid contributing to denial by "soft pedaling" the severity of the situation, e.g., by telling a newly diagnosed patient that he or she has "borderline diabetes," "mild diabetes," or "a touch of sugar" or telling a patient with poor metabolic control that he or she is "doing OK." This approach may lead the patient to believe that diabetes is not serious and effective management is not important.

Clinicians also should avoid the opposite approach, describing diabetes and its potential consequences in devastating terms, because that also can contribute to maladaptive denial, especially for a patient who already is using denial to cope with excessive fear. Fear-inducing communication may lead the patient to increase denial to manage this fear. Thus, clinicians should make sure they know which scenario they are dealing with before choosing an information-giving strategy. Careful questioning, as described in Chapters 1 and 21, can be helpful in this regard.

To avoid maladaptive denial, patients need information directed to meeting their specific situations. If patients are using denial to cope with fear, help them focus on how it is possible to dramatically reduce their chances of future complications by effective self-care. If patients' denial arises from a lack of concern, make sure they are aware of the seriousness of diabetes and the potential negative consequences of ineffective self-care. Once the proper emotional context has been established, help patients develop self-care skills to enable them to effectively manage their diabetes. Specific barriers may be addressed through formal diabetes education and nutritional counseling.

Address Fear and Hyper-Vigilance

Some patients, especially those with type 1 diabetes who engage in intensive management, may respond to fear with an obsessive preoccupation with tight control and compulsive efforts to achieve optimal glycemic control. This kind of behavior is the opposite of denial and may be thought of as too much of a good thing. When encouraging patients to implement effective self-care, be aware that this advice might fuel obsessive-compulsive tendencies in certain predisposed individuals.

It is often hard to draw the line between hyper-vigilance and effective intensive management. The best indicator is the comfort the patient feels with the regimen, especially if the regimen is an intensive one. Careful questioning is probably the best way to identify those whose approach to treatment is hyper-vigilant. Useful questions include, "How much do you worry about your blood glucose going high (or low)?" and "How strict are you about sticking to your regimen?" Patients with obsessive-compulsive tendencies may say they have to be perfect and engage in ritualistic behavior—to eat exactly the same amount at exactly the same time every day, to do many blood glucose tests every day, and to stick precisely to the regimen, even when it disrupts other aspects of life, such as social relationships, work, and family life.

The patient's comfort with his or her behavior is the key to understanding the behavior. Some people stick closely to schedules for diabetes-related activities and significantly adjust other aspects of their lives, yet do this without feeling driven. Good self-care *1)* focuses on the dual goals of maintaining good metabolic control and good quality of life, *2)* is flexible in the pursuit of these goals, and *3)* makes the diabetes regimen a matter-of-fact, albeit very important, part of life, not a painful preoccupation that dominates all other aspects of living.

Balance Physical and Emotional Well-Being

If a patient appears to be sacrificing quality of life for rigid regimen adherence, address the issue directly, emphasizing several guidelines for balancing the need to "do the right thing" with the equally important need to "live well." Extremes are unworkable, and finding a personally acceptable balance is the key to success. Perfection is unattainable even with the most heroic efforts, and an unbending effort to achieve perfection is a recipe for eventual breakdown. With effort and appropriate support and counseling, each person can find workable approaches to most diabetes-related situations, no matter how difficult or impossible it seems at first.

BE AWARE THAT ANGER AND ACTING OUT ARE COMMON RESPONSES

Anger is another emotion that may be seen in patients with diabetes. This anger may be based on the belief that diabetes represents an unfair and unbearable burden. Intense anger may preclude an effective approach to identifying the changes that are necessary to successfully live with diabetes. Anger may present as a "who cares" attitude, extreme risk-taking, or overt hostility.

Anger is especially problematic for the patient-clinician relationship because clinicians may unconsciously feel that the anger is directed at them. Indeed, often patients will be addressing the clinician when expressing their anger. This expressed anger can lead the clinician to feel anxious and want to terminate the interaction. This is a natural response. Unfortunately, it can result in a dismissive attitude, minimizing the patient's problems because it is unpleasant to deal with them (see Chapter 3).

Acknowledge the Patient's Anger

The key to effectively managing a patient's anger is to acknowledge it and work with it. Joining with the patient validates the emotion as a step toward resolving it. Encourage patients to express their anger and to identify specific aspects of living with diabetes that make them angry. This puts the patient and provider on the "same side of the fence" and helps focus their joint efforts on the problems to be addressed. Joining with the patient in this fashion helps overcome divisiveness by removing the clinician from the path of the anger and is liberating for both patient and clinician.

Address the Cause of Anger

Anger arises at least partly because of one or more burdens. A patient may be angry because of the belief that certain restrictions must be endured, e.g., giving up a particular food or activity. Usually, it is possible to work with the patient to develop a less restrictive plan without compromising metabolic control. For example, a patient could eat a favorite food occasionally or adjust medication to compensate for an activity. Once past the issue of dealing with an angry patient, it is possible to work together on finding a solution—one that will allow the patient to take better care of his or her diabetes.

Clinicians should be aware that patients who experience excessive anger are at elevated risk for depression (see Chapter 22). Whereas these emotions seem at opposite extremes (anger as an intense emotion, depression as a flat affect), they are better seen as emotion turned outward (anger) or inward (depression). Anger may serve as a source of emotional energy that, when exhausted, results in emotional collapse. Or patients may alternate between anger and depression. Clinicians should recognize the risk of anger masking depression and be prepared to deal with the depression when it emerges.

BE AWARE THAT GUILT AND RECRIMINATION ARE COMMON RESPONSES

Guilt is another common emotion in diabetes, and often results in recrimination. Patients may blame themselves for the onset of their diabetes, e.g., "if only I had not eaten so many sweets," or more realistically, "if only I had not put on so much weight." Parents of children with diabetes may blame themselves for their child's misfortune. Spouses may feel responsible for a patient's poor control or recent complications. However, guilt is rarely a useful emotional response.

Help Transform Guilt Into Motivation

It may be useful to try to alleviate guilt, but it is important not to get in an argument with the person experiencing guilt. These arguments can result when the clinician attempts to minimize the guilt, leading the patient to argue even more forcefully for his or her culpability. While guilt itself is not useful, it contains a useful kernel of recognition—a knowledge that behavior can make a difference. The key is to get the person to focus on what can be done in the future rather than what may or may not have been done in the past. If the patient's behavior has influenced how things have come out so far, it should be possible to change the future by changing his or her behavior. Therefore, it is important to help the person see that it is possible to change his or her behavior and future. Rebuilding the patient's self-efficacy and identifying potentially effective behavioral solutions are mutually reinforcing and can lead to improved physical and emotional well-being.

BE AWARE THAT DEPRESSION AND ANXIETY DISORDERS ARE COMMON

An emotional problem may be so severe that it represents a diagnosable disorder in its own right. For example, a person may be so sad and grief-stricken that he or she is clinically depressed. Depression and anxiety disorders are more common in patients with diabetes and can severely hamper medical management of diabetes. Feelings of hopelessness and helplessness often associated with depression may contribute to a cycle of poor self-care, worsened glycemia, and deepened depression. In addition, the natural course of depression may be more devastating in patients who have diabetes than in individuals who have no medical problems; depressive episodes may occur more frequently, be more severe, and last longer. For more on depression and diabetes, see Chapter 22.

It is important to identify depression when it is present and to provide effective treatment. Unfortunately, the task of diagnosing depression in patients with diabetes can be problematic because many common physical symptoms of depression (insomnia, fatigue, appetite disturbances, and decreased libido) also are symptoms of hyperglycemia. Because many people with diabetes are hyperglycemic at diagnosis, the presence of affective symptoms—guilt, anhedonia (markedly diminished interest or pleasure in almost all activities), feelings of helplessness or worthlessness, memory impairment, and indecision—is particularly useful for an accurate diagnosis.

Some symptoms of anxiety disorder are similar to those of depression. These include fatigue, sleep disturbance, difficulty concentrating, and irritability. Other symptoms of anxiety disorder include restlessness and muscle tension. As with depression, some symptoms of anxiety disorder overlap with those of metabolic dysregulation, but, in this case, they overlap with symptoms of hypoglycemia.

REFER PATIENTS TO MENTAL HEALTH PROFESSIONALS WHEN APPROPRIATE

Sometimes, the clinician may feel that dealing with emotional responses to diabetes is not possible because of the severity of the problem and limits in available time or skill. Under these circumstances, it is important to have a mental health referral source. Psychosocial treatment is a specialty in its own right. Try to identify a mental health specialist who has experience in treating people with diabetes. If such a person is not available, consider one who has experience treating patients with other chronic diseases or one who is interested in treating people with diabetes.

CONCLUSION

The painful emotions noted above need to be respected. Acknowledge these emotions and your own reaction to them, and address the situation before attempting to teach diabetes management. Open-ended questions concerning diabetes-related feelings may help some patients recognize and acknowledge their emotions. The beliefs that underlie these emotions also must be addressed. Let the patient know that adjustment to living with diabetes can be difficult. Take advantage of "teachable moments" (i.e., situations when motivation is high) to reinforce the patient's efforts to deal with the emotional and practical aspects of life with diabetes.

The patient's family is an essential source of support. Include them whenever possible (see Chapter 19). Refer patients to support groups, and offer recommendations for periodical literature, videotapes, pamphlets, and books that deal with the emotional side of diabetes. Finally, encourage patients to join the American Diabetes Association and other organizations whose activities may facilitate acceptance.

Effectively dealing with a chronic disease such as diabetes requires a special kind of patient-clinician relationship. It is important for clinicians to help patients deal with emotional barriers to self-care. These barriers, which range from emotions of fear, anger, and guilt to disorders of anxiety and depression, and coping strategies of denial, catastrophizing, hyper-vigilance, and acting out, will be different for different individuals. Be sensitive to the existence of emotional responses to diabetes and take active steps to help patients resolve any problematic responses.

BIBLIOGRAPHY

Hamburg BA, Inhoff GE: Coping with predictable crises of diabetes. *Diabetes Care* 6:409–416, 1983

Peyrot M, Rubin RR: Psychosocial aspects of diabetes care. In *Diabetes: Clinical Science in Practice.* Leslie D, Robbins D, Eds. Cambridge, U.K., Cambridge University Press, 1995, p. 465–477

Rubin RR, Peyrot M: Psychosocial problems and interventions in diabetes. *Diabetes Care* 15:1640–1657, 1991

Mark Peyrot, PhD, is Chair of the Department of Sociology and Director of the Center for Social and Community Research at Loyola College in Baltimore, MD.

21

Understanding and Treating Patients with Diabetes Burnout

WILLIAM H. POLONSKY, PhD, CDE

Mrs. J is a 54-year-old secretary with a 6-year history of type 2 diabetes. Frightened by the possibility of long-term complications, she has always been anxious about managing her diabetes as well as possible. She was relatively successful in the first months after diagnosis, but she became increasingly frustrated with her prescribed meal plan, which she found quite restrictive, and with her inability to establish a regular schedule for daily walking. Despite her best efforts, she was unable to lose weight as directed (partly because of her new oral hypoglycemic agent) and experienced several frightening episodes of mild hypoglycemia. Over the years, her attempts at self-management have slowly deteriorated. At this time, she continues to take her oral medication faithfully each day, but she tests her blood glucose only rarely (approximately once a week). As she notes, "Why bother testing at all? It's always too high!" She continues to follow her prescribed meal plan, at least through the early parts of the day. By suppertime, however, she begins to binge, which continues unchecked until bedtime. Regular physical activity is no longer even attempted. Her husband and close friends are constantly pushing her to "try harder," but this has not been helpful and has only increased her sense of isolation with diabetes. She tries not to think about her illness and avoids seeing her physician, who she fears will recommend that she begin insulin. When she does think about diabetes, she feels angry and frustrated with herself, feeling overwhelmed, exhausted, and defeated by her diabetes and very worried about her future health. Mrs. J is suffering from diabetes burnout.

WHAT IS DIABETES BURNOUT?

Burnout was originally conceptualized as a common response to a chronically difficult and frustrating job, where the individual works harder and harder each day and yet has little sense that these actions are making a real difference. The individual may feel chronically overextended and depleted, and there may be a sense of inadequacy or guilt that he or she is failing at the job. Feelings of helplessness, hopelessness, irritability, and hostility are also common, resulting in a state of chronic emotional exhaustion.

As in Mrs. J's case, the experience of living with diabetes may commonly lead to similar feelings of burnout. The patient may come to feel that the day-to-day vigilance and effort needed to properly manage diabetes is too burdensome and frustrating and the results too inconsequential to make the effort worthwhile. Feeling overwhelmed and defeated by diabetes, the patient may worry that he or she is not taking care of the diabetes well enough and yet feel unable, unmotivated, or unwilling to change. At its roots, diabetes burnout is about hopelessness and poor self-efficacy, i.e., the patient's sense that he or she cannot achieve and/or maintain appropriate diabetes self-care, even while believing it to be an important goal. Not surprisingly, diabetes burnout often overlaps with depression, which is known to be common in patients with diabetes (see Chapter 22).

WHY WORRY ABOUT DIABETES BURNOUT?

While the prevalence of diabetes burnout is not yet known, we suspect that it may be relatively common. In recent studies, we found that diabetes-specific emotional distress was widespread among patients at several large medical clinics across the United States, with approximately 60–70% of the patients sampled reporting at least one serious diabetes-related concern. Many, but not all, patients who report higher levels of diabetes burnout (chronic frustration and feelings of failure) have markedly higher glycated hemoglobin A1C (A1C) levels and report significantly poorer self-care.

Diabetes burnout may be even more prevalent in patients who have dropped out of medical care. These patients may have compromised their diabetes self-care such that chronically poor metabolic control results, increasing the likelihood of serious long-term complications. Tragically, health care providers may see many of these patients only rarely until complications begin to emerge. We suspect that future research will document that diabetes burnout is a major risk factor for poor metabolic control and the consequent, perhaps early, onset of long-term diabetes complications. If diabetes burnout can be identified, understood, and treated in clinic populations and, hopefully, in harder-to-reach populations, we believe that this could potentially contribute to improving long-term metabolic control and reducing rates of long-term complications in a substantial subgroup of patients.

KNOW THE SIX STRATEGIES FOR ALLEVIATING DIABETES BURNOUT

To alleviate diabetes burnout and assist patients in maintaining better self-care, six major strategies are recommended. These strategies are somewhat overlapping and may be considered to be additive in their efficacy.

Learn to Recognize Diabetes Burnout

Assessment of diabetes burnout can be difficult because patients may be unable to recognize their own complex feelings about diabetes or may feel embarrassed to discuss their feelings with health care providers, whom they may perceive (rightly or wrongly) as judgmental. Make patients comfortable in being honest about the aggravation and distress that often accompany diabetes self-care by normalizing self-care problems. For example, rather than asking, "You're not having any problems with managing your diabetes, are you?," consider saying, "Everyone struggles with managing their diabetes from time to time. What's that struggle like for you?' or "Can you tell me about some of the things that are driving you crazy about diabetes these days?" (see Chapter 1).

A patient with diabetes burnout may have any of the following signs or symptoms:

- Feels that diabetes is controlling (or trying to control) his or her life.
- Feels overwhelmed by self-care goals and actions and usually feels that he or she is failing with diabetes.
- Has strong, negative feelings about diabetes.
- Feels alone with diabetes and feels that no one understands.
- Admits to chronically poor self-care and poor glycemic control (brief episodes of excellent control may also occur).
- Has seen health care providers infrequently and may have no record of regular, ongoing care.
- Reports strong ambivalence about improving self-care (may feel that proper self-management is not worth the effort, but feels guilty and/or frightened about his or her history of poor self-care).

Establish a Strong, Collaborative Relationship With Patients

Patients with diabetes burnout often anticipate an adversarial relationship with their health care provider, feeling certain that they will be judged, demeaned, and/or treated disrespectfully. Thus, they may be somewhat withdrawn or avoidant during sessions, and they may tend to postpone, cancel, or altogether avoid appointments with health care providers (see Chapter 2). Such feelings and expectations may not be totally unreasonable given that these patients may have had previous negative interactions with significant others (including health care providers) about their diabetes. To intervene effectively, it is essential to be respectful of the patient's struggle with diabetes self-care. Clearly delineate the areas of responsibility for the patient, clarifying that the provider can serve as an advisor only, and strongly encourage active patient participation in all decision-making, goal-setting, and problem-solving. It is important to avoid an overly authoritarian or parental attitude (see Chapter 1 on empowerment). Focus on promoting subjective adherence (the patient's own interest in reaching a desired treatment goal) rather than objective compliance (the patient's obedience to the provider's instructions). To encourage a collaborative relationship, even office geography may play a role. For example, sitting next to the patient, rather than behind a desk, may help to promote a less authoritarian relationship.

In a meeting with a diabetes burnout patient, take time to review all self-care behaviors. As goals are established (see below), remember to help the patient identify where he or she is successful, not just where self-care shortcomings may lie. Also, pay respectful attention to the patient's blood glucose records. No matter how meager such records may be, if the patient is able to prepare and share records, consider the records and discuss them with the patient. Indeed, giving thoughtful attention to records is such a considerate and respectful gesture toward all patients that it may be one of the best predictors of whether the patient continues to bring records to future sessions.

Because alleviating diabetes burnout is likely to take time, a supportive and concerned provider will be most effective when continuity of regular care and contact is established. As described earlier, the patient with diabetes burnout may tend to avoid or cancel appointments, especially when he or she is discouraged with self-care (e.g., "I've kept so few records that there's no need to go to my appointment; my doctor will just be angry with me anyway"). Thus, when the patient and provider can proactively schedule a series of regular visits over 6–12 months and there is a clearly stated agreement that the patient will attend these visits, regardless of his or her "success" at self-care, the patient is more likely to feel respected and cared about, feel that self-care is important, and feel that he or she is an important (and responsible) member of the health care team.

At first, the less time between scheduled visits, the better. And, when at all possible, follow-up contacts between visits (e.g., phone calls, faxing of patient blood glucose records, provider letters, and reinforcing comments to the patient) are valuable. One patient, for example, stated that the most important factor in ending her years of diabetes burnout was one particular action of her new physician. Between her first and second visit, he phoned her several times (once a week) to check on her progress. By this unique action alone, she began to feel cared about and respected, and, subsequently, she began to care more about herself and her diabetes.

Negotiate Patient-Centered Goals

When self-care goals are unclear and/or unreasonable, diabetes burnout is more likely to occur. Help patients identify their current expectations and assist them in developing new self-care goals that are concrete, achievable, and of personal interest to them (see Chapter 6).

Mrs. J, for example, had been told that walking each day was absolutely essential for her diabetes management. While she enjoyed walking, she had no clear sense of how many miles were necessary to be successful, and she slowly but surely began to convince herself that she was "failing" every day (she was averaging 1 mile, 4 days a week). After further discussion, she realized that she had somehow decided that the minimum for "successful" walking was 3 miles, 7 days a week. To prevent her from giving up her walking program completely (which she was close to doing), the provider assisted her in selecting a target for weekly walking that was more reasonable for her (1 mile, 5 days a week), a goal that helped her to feel successful and upon which she could gradually build more challenging goals. To promote "success experiences," diabetes self-care goals must be concrete, specific, time-limited, uncomplicated, measurable, and—most importantly—realistic.

Pay Attention to Strong Negative Feelings About Diabetes

In diabetes burnout, goal planning and other behavioral interventions are not likely to be successfully implemented when the patient is so guilt-ridden, despondent, angry, or fearful about diabetes that he or she does not feel hopeful that such actions will be valuable. Take time to hear and acknowledge the patient's difficult feelings about diabetes (see Chapter 20). Toward this end, it is essential to put aside preconceived notions about how the patient may feel, and make sure to ask directly about diabetes-related distress (e.g., "How is diabetes aggravating you?") and to ascertain how the patient makes sense of diabetes (e.g., "How do you feel about having diabetes?," "Do you think taking care of your diabetes is worth doing?," or "Are you worried about the possibility of complications?"). In addition, listening well and respectfully, rather than leaping quickly to find solutions for the patient's feelings, may be the most important step toward change. The provider's most important response should be to normalize the patient's negative feelings about diabetes, reassuring the patient that such feelings are common and understandable. In the course of such discussions, however, careful attention to the possibility of a more pervasive problem that may necessitate an appropriate referral, such as a depressive disorder, is critical.

Optimize Social Support

The patient with diabetes burnout may feel quite isolated with diabetes, believing that no one understands or appreciates the struggle with the illness. Diabetes burnout may begin to dissipate when the patient begins to feel supported—when a friend, family member, or health care provider truly understands and actively roots for him or her (see Chapter 19). To promote more valuable support, there are three major problem-solving interventions to use: *1*) add positive support behaviors, *2*) eliminate negative support behaviors, and *3*) clarify regimen responsibilities.

First, ask the patient to consider the idiosyncratic ways, no matter how silly, selfish, or unrealistic these may seem at first, in which family and friends might be of more direct assistance in managing diabetes. This assistance includes emotional as well as behavioral support. Assist the patient in selecting one of those desired behaviors, choosing who they might want to approach for support, and determining how they might go about asking in a tactful and considerate manner.

While the patient may benefit by thinking of creative ways in which to ask friends and family to help, he or she may also profit by considering those ongoing behaviors of significant others that are not helpful and need to be stopped. Diabetes burnout may be more likely when the patient's spouse downplays the difficulty and importance of diabetes care, demanding, for example, that cookies and candy be available in the house for all other family members and telling the patient to "just use willpower" to avoid these sweets. Also, friends, family, and health care providers may serve as "diabetes police," choosing to "help" the patient manage diabetes, regardless of whether the patient may want such assistance. When the patient feels hounded by such infantilizing comments as "You shouldn't be eating that," "You seem upset; maybe you should check your blood sugar," or "If you want to lose weight, you better start applying more self-discipline," the patient may begin to withdraw from significant others, becoming more isolated and discouraged. By encouraging the patient to confront significant others, in as creative and tactful a manner as possible, and by finding ways to redirect loved ones' "helpfulness" into more beneficial actions (see Chapter 19 on involving families), self-care may improve and diabetes burnout may be significantly reduced. For example, Mrs. J asked her husband to stop constantly recommending that she "try harder" and, instead, requested that he join her in regular evening activities that might distract her from binge eating (e.g., a walk through the neighborhood).

Finally, consider the potential value of a family meeting, especially when there is apparent confusion about who is responsible for each self-care activity.

Engage Patients in Active Problem-Solving

When considering an intervention for a patient with diabetes burnout, consider these four major aspects of problem-solving.

1. Because feeling overwhelmed is a central facet of diabetes burnout, the provider will need to help the patient to prioritize the self-care changes he or she may be willing to make and then carefully limit any planned regimen changes to one self-care behavior at a time (as demonstrated in the discussion above, this practice increases the likelihood of a "success experience"). For example, Mr. F, a 39-year-old man with type 1 diabetes, decided that, after years of diabetes burnout and very poor self-care, he was ready to begin managing his diabetes "perfectly" (i.e., making major changes in his eating, exercise, frequency of blood sugar monitoring, insulin usage, and more). Rather than support such a large and rapid change of behavior, the provider encouraged the patient to start with only one selected change before moving on to his other goals (see Chapter 6).

2. Any planned change in self-care, especially if it involves a behavior that has not been a routine part of the patient's lifestyle, should initially focus on building that behavior into a regularly established habit. For Mr. F, who chose to begin with regular blood glucose monitoring, this was certain to be an important area of concern, because over the past 5 years, he had tested his blood glucose levels on a very irregular basis (approximately once a month). Thus, the focus of the initial intervention was solving how he could begin monitoring regularly pre-breakfast, including how he would remember to do so (e.g., what other morning event he could link his monitoring to) as well as how he would make sure to have the time available each morning (e.g., setting his alarm to arise 10 min earlier each morning).

3. As possible solutions to a problem are considered, keep in mind the patient's previous successes with a similar problem. For example, in the previous year, Mr. F had succeeded in restructuring his morning ritual so that he would remember to take his vitamins at breakfast (he placed the vitamins next to the coffeepot). He adapted this solution to successfully establish the habit of morning blood glucose monitoring (he placed his meter and supplies next to his shaving kit).
4. Consider simple environmental solutions first. These solutions tend to be the easiest to adopt. Mr. F could have been encouraged to use his "willpower" to remember his monitoring each morning, but he was more likely to be successful if he followed his clinician's suggestions for simple concrete adjustments in his environment (e.g., leave your meter next to your shaving kit, and set your alarm 10 min earlier).

CONCLUSION

Diabetes can be a difficult and burdensome illness, and feelings of distress are common. When the negative consequences of diabetes self-care are perceived as too burdensome, diabetes burnout may result. Diabetes burnout is characterized by feelings of being overwhelmed and defeated by diabetes, a sense of hopelessness that appropriate diabetes self-care cannot be achieved and/or maintained, and, consequently, poor self-care and chronically elevated blood glucose levels. We suspect that a substantial subgroup of patients may be suffering (albeit silently) from diabetes burnout. Therefore, proper identification and treatment of diabetes burnout may be very important. Six major strategies for treating diabetes burnout were presented. It is hoped that future research will point to a more refined description of diabetes burnout, better evidence as to the actual prevalence and consequences of diabetes burnout, and a more comprehensive (and experimentally rigorous) set of treatment strategies.

BIBLIOGRAPHY

Greenfield S, Kaplan SH, Ware JE, Yano EM, Frank HJL: Patients' participation in medical care: effects on blood sugar control and quality of life in diabetes. *J Gen Intern Med* 3:448–457, 1988

Hoover JW: Patient 'burnout' can explain non-compliance. In *World Book of Diabetes in Practice*. Vol. 3. Krall LP, Ed. New York, Elsevier Science Publishers, 1988

Polonsky WH: *Diabetes Burnout: What To Do When You Can't Take It Anymore*. Alexandria, VA, American Diabetes Association, 1999

Polonsky WH, Anderson BJ, Lohrer PA, Welch G, Jacobson AM, Schwartz C: Assessment of diabetes-specific distress. *Diabetes Care* 18:754–760, 1995

Polonsky WH, Welch GM: Listening to our patients' concerns: understanding and addressing diabetes-specific emotional distress. *Diabetes Spectrum* 9:8–11, 1996

Rollnick S, Mason P, Butler C: *Health Behavior Change*. New York, Churchill Livingstone, 1999

Rubin RR, Biermann J, Toohey B: *Psyching Out Diabetes*. 3rd ed. Los Angeles, CA, Lowell House, 1999

Strowig SM, Basco M, Cercone S: A cognitive behavioral approach to diabetes management. *Diabetes Spectrum* 7:341–342, 1994

William H. Polonsky, PhD, CDE, is an Assistant Clinical Professor in Psychiatry at the University of California, San Diego in La Jolla, CA.

22

Recognizing and Managing Depression in Patients with Diabetes

PATRICK J. LUSTMAN, PhD,
PUNEET K. SINGH, BA, AND RAY E. CLOUSE, MD

The term "depression" denotes two distinctly different experiences. The first is the common experience: occasional periods of feeling down, irritable, stressed, or just generally out-of-sorts. These depressed feelings are usually short-lived and inconsequential. A bad day is followed by a good day, and life goes on. The second is the experience of depression as a serious, sometimes life-threatening mental disorder. This depression is conferred the status of a medical diagnosis called major depressive disorder. The disorder presents as a cluster of mental (e.g., sadness, loss of interest) and physical (e.g., fatigue, sleep difficulties) symptoms that persist over an extended period of time and significantly impair interpersonal behavior, occupational functioning, and quality of life. In this chapter, the term depression is used as a synonym for this severe form of depression.

UNDERSTAND THE FREQUENCY, CAUSES, AND CONSEQUENCES OF DEPRESSION IN DIABETES

Patients with diabetes are twice as likely to suffer from depression as those without diabetes. The psychiatric disorder is present in ~15% of patients with diabetes and is equally common in those with either type 1 or type 2 diabetes. The rate of depression is significantly higher in women than in men with diabetes, reflecting the sex difference observed in studies of the general U.S. population. The fact that depression is more common in people with diabetes does not prove that diabetes causes depression or that depression causes diabetes. Rather, the frequent co-occurrence of depression and diabetes establishes that these conditions will have many opportunities to affect one another.

The cause of depression in people with diabetes is presently unknown but is probably complex, resulting from an interaction among psychological, physical, and genetic factors. The precise contribution of these factors will vary from patient to patient. Diabetes is a demanding condition, and adjusting to dietary restrictions, treatment regimens, hospitalizations, and increased financial obligations can be stressful for patients and their loved ones. Coping with limitations in function associated with advancing diabetes, such as loss of vision or sexual capacity, is difficult and may contribute to depression. Various physical changes associated with diabetes, including neurochemical and neurovascular abnormalities, may also be causal factors. Lastly, research has shown that genetic factors unrelated to diabetes may cause depression in patients with diabetes.

Whatever the cause, once present, depression can interact negatively with diabetes. The pervasive nature of the psychiatric disorder's adverse effects is striking. Depression has direct and indirect links to both poor glycemic control and diabetes complications (see Chapter 20). A model of the interactions is shown in Figure 22.1 and discussed below. At the epicenter of the model, depression intersects with every other box. It has been directly associated with poor glycemic control, the major cause of diabetes complications. In addition, depression indirectly promotes poor glycemic control through its contributions to obesity, physical inactivity, and treatment nonadherence.

As could be expected from its effects on glycemic control, depression is linked to complications of diabetes. A recent meta-analysis established an association of depression with increased occurrence of neuropathy, nephropathy, retinopathy, and macrovascular disease. The association is not simply that depression occurs as a reaction to the hardships of advancing disease. Several prospective studies in adults with diabetes demonstrate that depression increases the incidence and hastens the onset of coronary heart disease, especially in women. Factors that can exacerbate diabetes complications, such as smoking, substance abuse, and insulin resistance, have also been correlated with depression. More-

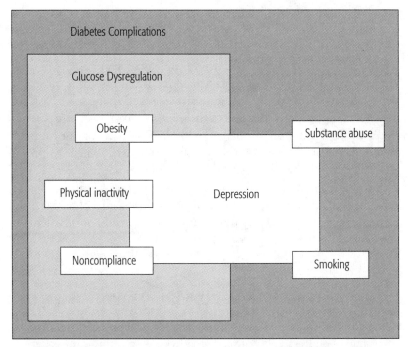

FIGURE 22.1 Depression has been associated with many behavioral and medical factors in patients with diabetes. Both depression and its associated factors have been linked to glucose dysregulation and diabetes complications. Intersecting boxes in this figure indicate significant associations proven in diabetes research. Adapted from Lustman PJ (Guest Editor): Depression in diabetes. *Diabetes Spectrum* 7:161–189, 1994.

over, depressed patients respond poorly to lifestyle interventions (e.g., smoking cessation and weight loss programs), further jeopardizing efforts to control diabetes and improve outcomes (see Chapters 9 and 10). Studies like these, as well as those that show depression promotes poor glycemic control, suggest that keeping patients free of depression could prevent or delay diabetes complications.

Depression affects perceptual processes and is thought to make people more sensitive to, and intolerant of, physical symptoms. For example, neuropathy pain that is normally an intermittent annoyance may feel constant and unbearable during a period of depression and prompt a visit to the physician. Depression even influences the reporting of symptoms that are usually considered exclusively physical manifestations of diabetes. Research has shown that gastrointestinal and autonomic as well as hyperglycemic and hypoglycemic symptoms are more often related to depression than to the biomedical processes presumed to produce them.

Thus, in addition to its effects on mood, functioning, interpersonal relationships, and quality of life, depression has added relevance in individuals with diabetes. It can accentuate medical symptoms, promote poor glycemic control and insulin resistance, and increase the risk for diabetes complications. Because of these interactions, certain aspects of the clinical presentation in a patient with diabetes may suggest the presence of depression. Depression should be considered *1*) when symptoms of hyperglycemia or hypoglycemia persist in the face of objective evidence of adequate glycemic control, *2*) when other symptoms lack a solid medical explanation or are out of proportion to the objective findings, *3*) when sexual dysfunction is raised as a concern, or *4*) whenever chronic pain is a dominant complaint.

IDENTIFY DEPRESSION IN INDIVIDUALS WITH DIABETES

Using currently accepted psychiatric diagnostic techniques, the diagnosis of major depressive disorder is made when a number of criterion symptoms occur together, are severe, and persist daily over a period of at least 2 weeks (Table 22.1). Sad mood or a significant loss of interest or pleasure are the *sine qua non* for the diagnosis, and one of these must be present along with any four of the other listed symptoms. The symptoms must be the source of significant distress or decline in social, occupational, or other important areas of functioning to count toward a diagnosis of depression. Criterion symptoms that result from taking medication or illicit drugs or that are referable to bereavement are discounted.

Symptoms judged as being caused by a medical condition do not count toward the diagnosis. Because uncontrolled diabetes can cause some of the very symptoms typical of depression (e.g., fatigue, weight changes), the rule is useful and discourages overdiagnosis of the emotional disorder. The fact that diabetes does not directly produce the key diagnostic symptoms (sadness and loss of interest or pleasure) reduces the likelihood of a false-positive diagnosis, and the utility of conventional criteria in patients with diabetes has been established. In short, diabetes, even when uncontrolled, does not impair the clinician's ability to easily and accurately diagnose depression.

TABLE 22.1   Diagnostic Criteria for Major Depressive Disorder

1. One of the following:
   • Depressed mood
   • Markedly diminished interest or pleasure in almost all activities

2. Four of the following:
   • Significant weight loss or gain
   • Insomnia or hypersomnia
   • Psychomotor agitation or retardation
   • Fatigue, loss of energy
   • Feelings of worthlessness or guilt
   • Impaired concentration or indecisiveness
   • Recurrent thoughts of death or suicide

3. Symptoms must be present most of the day.

4. Symptoms must be present nearly daily for ≥2 weeks.

5. Symptoms must be the result of significant distress or impairment and not be attributable to medications, medical conditions, or bereavement.

All five criteria are required.

Despite its relevance to the course of diabetes, depression is recognized and treated in less than one-third of all diabetic cases. Many factors contribute to this problem, including the assumption that depression is merely secondary to diabetes and not of independent importance. The perception persists despite clear evidence that depression may interact negatively with diabetes, and it unfortunately serves to focus clinical management efforts exclusively on the medical condition.

Depression in the medically ill also may go unrecognized because clinicians generally do not have the time and training required to perform formal psychodiagnostic interviews. Brief paper and pencil screening instruments capable of detecting depression can help with this problem. These instruments are well suited to the realities of making psychiatric diagnoses in outpatient medical settings. For example, the 21-item Beck Depression Inventory (BDI) does not require an interview, is self-administered, takes 5–10 min to complete, and is scored easily and manually by summing the ratings for each of the 21 items.

We recommend that patients with depression symptoms lasting ≥2 weeks and BDI scores ≥16 undergo formal diagnostic testing to determine whether major depressive disorder is present. This cutoff score captures >70% of the patients with depression. In situations where resources are more plentiful and the emphasis is on not overlooking depression cases, the BDI cutoff score could be lowered to 12, a score that would capture at least 90% of patients with diagnosable depression.

KNOW ABOUT THE COURSE AND MANAGEMENT OF DEPRESSION IN DIABETES

Depression in diabetes is a recurring condition in which periods of sadness alternate with periods of feeling normal or well. On average, afflicted patients suffer one episode annually throughout their lifetimes. Without treatment directed specifically at depression, individual episodes do not rapidly remit of their own accord and are not responsive to efforts focused solely on improving glycemic control.

There are two general methods for treating depression: one is medication and the other is psychotherapy. Psychotherapy differs from general supportive counseling in its application of a specific set of proven techniques aimed at removing depression symptoms and improving psychosocial functioning. In general, medication and psychotherapy are equally effective treatments for depression, and ~50–60% of treated patients will achieve a remission within 3 months. There is evidence that some patients may benefit from the combination of medication and psychotherapy, but little information is available to guide the clinician in selecting patients for this approach. Initial treatment is often predetermined by the patient's selection of a mental health professional. Primary care physicians and diabetologists are most likely to treat depression with medication and common-sense advice. Psychologists and social workers use counseling and formal psychotherapy. Psychiatrists may use a combination of these treatments but generally emphasize medication.

Consideration of the individual's symptom picture provides a logical basis for effective treatment planning. The first choice of treatment for depression dominated by somatic symptoms might be medication, whereas psychotherapy would be a well-chosen treatment for depression characterized by interpersonal difficulties. Psychotherapy is also the treatment of choice for patients who want to learn coping or self-management techniques aimed at removing depression and preventing its recurrence. Medication is more appropriate for patients who do not have the time or financial resources for psychotherapy or who are simply not inclined to talk about their problems. The presence of suicidal ideation requires access to the full range of depression treatments, and suicidal patients are most often referred to a psychiatrist. Additional thought must be given to the impact of treatment on the medical disease. For example, one class of antidepressant medication might be more desirable than another for a diabetic patient with heart disease or bowel dysfunction.

Antidepressant agents commonly used to treat depression along with dosage and side effects are shown in Table 22.2. These medications are equal in their antidepressant effects when used in primary care settings and psychiatric clinics, and the same is presumed in diabetic samples. Consequently, selection is based on such factors as presenting symptoms, coexisting medical conditions, drug interactions, and side effects. The conventional tricyclic antidepressants have been used effectively in primary care for >40 years and are particularly helpful in regulating sleep. When prescribing these agents, clinicians should consider the potential for weight gain, anticholinergic side effects, orthostatic hypotension, and other adverse cardiovascular effects. Tricyclic antidepressants may also worsen glycemic control in some patients. A recent clinical trial showed that nortriptyline was effective in treating depression but had an adverse, hyperglycemic impact that was unrelated to the medication's effect on weight.

Hyperglycemia has not been reported in patients treated with the selective serotonin reuptake inhibitors and other newer antidepressants. In fact, these agents appear to improve glycemic control, as was seen in a recent trial using fluoxetine. Selective serotonin reuptake inhibitors are at least as effective as tricyclic antidepressants in treating depression and do not usually cause weight gain or sedation. Potential benefits must be balanced against the possibility of gastrointestinal distress, agitation, and sexual dysfunction. Monoamine oxidase inhibitors and electroconvulsive therapy are usually only considered for severe depression that does not respond to the treatment described above.

Psychotherapy occupies a uniquely important role in the treatment of depression because, unlike medication, it has no physical side effects contraindicating its use in diabetes. Cognitive behavior therapy (CBT) and interpersonal therapy (IPT) are psychotherapeutic treatments with proven antidepressant efficacy. CBT evolved from observations that depressed people think in stereotypic ways ("I hate myself, my life stinks, and I have no future"). Depression is removed by teaching

TABLE 22.2 Selected Antidepressant Medications, Dosage, and Side Effects

Drug	Usual therapeutic dose (mg/day)	Side effect†						
		Anticholinergic*	Central nervous system‡		Cardiovascular		Other	
			Drowsiness	Insomnia/ agitation	Orthostatic hypotension	Cardiac arrhythmia	Gastrointestinal distress	Weight gain (>6 kg)
Tricyclics								
Amitriptyline	150–200	4	4	0	4	3	1	4
Desipramine	150–200	1	1	1	2	2	1	1
Imipramine	150–200	3	3	1	4	3	1	3
Nortriptyline	75–100	1	1	0	2	2	1	1
Heterocyclics								
Bupropion	200–300	0	0	2	0	1	1	0
Trazodone	200–300	0	4	0	2	1	1	1
Newer antidepressants								
Fluoxetine	20	0	1	2	0	0	3	0
Paroxetine	20	2	1	2	0	0	3	0
Sertraline	50–150	0	1	2	0	0	3	0
Venlafaxine§	75–225	0	1	2	1	0	3	0
Nefazodone	200–300	0	1	0	1	0	3	0

Adapted from U.S. Department of Health and Human Services, Agency for Health Care Policy and Research, *Depression Guideline Panel: Depression in Primary Care: Volume 2. Treatment of Major Depression* (Clinical Practice Guidelines, no. 5). Washington, DC, U.S. Government Printing Office (AHCPR publ. no. 93-0551), 1993, and from Lustman PJ, Clouse RE, Alrakawi A, Rubin E, Gelenberg AJ: Treatment of major depression in adults with diabetes: a primary care perspective. *Clinical Diabetes* 15:122–126, 1997.

*Includes dry mouth, blurred vision, urinary hesitancy, and constipation.

† Relative occurrence of side effects among agents listed: ranked from 0 (absent or rare) to 4 (relatively common).

‡ A reduction of seizure threshold can occur with all antidepressants and is most pronounced with bupropion.

§ Unlike the selective serotonin reuptake inhibitors, venlafaxine at higher doses can cause an elevation of diastolic blood pressure.

patients to identify, challenge, and replace depressing thought patterns. IPT views depression as arising in an interpersonal context in which stressful and conflicted relationships are thought to cause, maintain, and exacerbate depression. Treatment involves the teaching of specific communication and social skills. This therapy may be particularly relevant in diabetes because changes in roles and functioning occur frequently as the medical disease worsens. Since CBT and IPT teach skills that help patients better cope with stressful life circumstances, both of these methods can help remove depression as well as prevent its recurrence (see Chapter 6). Like other antidepressant treatment, psychotherapy can also improve glycemic control. One study showed that depressed patients treated with CBT had significantly better glycemic control than untreated patients 6 months after completing treatment.

The potential effect of a specific treatment on existing medical conditions is just one factor to consider in managing depression. A multitude of logistic, financial, and personal issues may also affect choice of depression treatment. For example, what is the patient's preference for treatment? A therapeutic alliance and increased adherence is best established when patients are involved in the treatment process. Does age, physical mobility, or mental acuity restrict treatment options? Does the patient's employment or lifestyle allow time for treatment? What are the patient's financial resources? Are medical and mental health professionals within easy access? In short, the patient's life circumstances can affect treatment selection.

CONCLUSION

Depression in people with diabetes is a prevalent and chronic condition. It has importance in diabetes that goes beyond its recognized effects on normal mental functioning. Depression will actually complicate the medical disease by influencing the reporting of diabetes symptoms, reducing adherence to medical therapy, promoting poor glycemic control, and increasing the risk of progressive end-organ damage. Brief paper and pencil tests like the BDI can be used in outpatient medical settings to screen for depression and help focus the health care team on patients in need of treatment. Treatment of depression is effective and important because of its positive effects on mood and quality of life, as well as its potential benefits to glycemic control and the reduction in diabetes complications.

ACKNOWLEDGMENTS

Work for this chapter was supported in part by grants DK-36452, DK-59364, and DK-53060 from the National Institutes of Health.

BIBLIOGRAPHY

Anderson RJ, Freedland KE, Clouse RE, Lustman PJ: The prevalence of comorbid depression in adults with diabetes: a meta-analysis. *Diabetes Care* 24:1069–1078, 2001

de Groot M, Anderson R, Freedland KE, Clouse RE, Lustman PJ: Association of depression and diabetes complications: a meta-analysis. *Psychosom Med* 63:619–630, 2001

Lustman PJ, Anderson RJ, Freedland KE, de Groot, MK, Carney RM, Clouse RE: Depression and poor glycemic control: a meta-analytic review of the literature. *Diabetes Care* 23:934–942, 2000

Lustman PJ, Clouse RE, Alrakawi A, Rubin E, Gelenberg AJ: Treatment of major depression in adults with diabetes: a primary care perspective. *Clinical Diabetes* 15:122–126, 1997

Lustman PJ, Griffith LS, Freedland KE, Kissel SS, Clouse RE: Cognitive behavior therapy for depression in type 2 diabetes: a randomized, controlled trial. *Ann Intern Med* 129:613–621, 1998

U.S. Department of Health and Human Services, Agency for Health Care Policy and Research, Depression Guideline Panel: *Depression in Primary Care: Volume 2. Treatment of Major Depression* (Clinical Practice Guidelines, no. 5). Washington, DC, U.S. Government Printing Office (AHCPR publ. no. 93-0551), 1993

Patrick J. Lustman, PhD, is a Professor of Psychiatry at Washington University School of Medicine in St. Louis, MO. Puneet K. Singh, BA, is a Research Associate in the Department of Psychiatry at Washington University School of Medicine in St. Louis, MO. Ray E. Clouse, MD, is a Professor of Medicine and Psychiatry at Washington University School of Medicine in St. Louis, MO.

23

Detecting and Treating Eating Disorders in Young Women with Type 1 Diabetes

ANN E. GOEBEL-FABBRI, PhD

Since early case reports in the 1980s, there has been considerable interest in examining the impact of type 1 diabetes on the development of eating disorders. Some researchers argue that the attention paid to food portions (especially carbohydrates), blood glucose levels, body weight, and exercise in standard medical treatment for type 1 diabetes parallels the rigid thinking about food and body image that is characteristic in women with eating disorders who do *not* also have diabetes. Results from the Diabetes Control and Complications Trial (DCCT) show that intensive insulin management of diabetes is associated with weight gain. Consequently, it may be that the very goals of state-of-the-art diabetes medical care increase the risk for developing an eating disorder.

Although research results are somewhat contradictory in this area, the most recent controlled studies suggest an increased risk of eating disorders among women with type 1 diabetes. For example, recent research shows that young women with diabetes have 2.4 times the risk of developing an eating disorder than age-matched women without diabetes. Studies that do *not* report higher rates of eating disorders in diabetes have typically not included insulin underdosing and insulin omission as part of the cluster of purging symptoms diagnostic for eating disorders.

Widespread, intermittent practice of strategic insulin omission and insulin underdosing for weight loss purposes have been reported among women with type 1 diabetes. This behavior is not limited to women who meet formal diagnostic criteria for eating disorders. One study found that out of a group of 341 women between the ages of 13 and 60 years, 31% reported intentional insulin omission. Rates of omission peaked in late adolescence and early adulthood. Insulin use and tighter blood glucose management caused significant distress for these women, with 44.3% reporting beliefs that taking insulin would cause weight gain and 35.9% reporting beliefs that tight blood glucose control would cause them to become fat.

For practitioners unfamiliar with direct care of people with eating disorders, an easy mistake is to believe that these are women who are "crazy," who are shallowly fixated on their outward appearance, or whose dieting has simply gotten a little too intensive. It is hard for some practitioners to understand why anyone with diabetes would intentionally misuse insulin for weight loss purposes when the medical risks associated with this behavior are so dangerous. The true nature of an eating disorder is difficult to grasp without a case example. The case described below is a composite of details from the experiences of many patients.

Case Example

Janelle is an 18-year-old high school senior who has had type 1 diabetes since age 10. Dr. Rich, her endocrinologist since diagnosis, noticed a pattern of elevated glycated hemoglobin A1C (A1C) levels accompanied by large weight fluctuations over the course of several years. Dr. Rich was concerned about Janelle's blood glucose and adherence to her diabetes management regimen. She suspected intentional insulin omission for weight loss, but Janelle denied this during their most recent medical encounter. Soon after the appointment, Janelle was hospitalized for diabetic ketoacidosis (DKA). Dr. Rich saw her for medical follow-up upon discharge and referred Janelle for a mental health evaluation by a psychologist familiar with issues related to diabetes.

Janelle denied that any problem existed at first, but she and the psychologist sat down together and reviewed her chart, looking at the blood glucose and weight patterns over time. Gradually, Janelle opened up about how terrible she felt gaining weight and how hard it was for her to grapple with unpredictable blood sugars during puberty. It took a few sessions for the full picture to emerge (Figure 23.1).

Here is Janelle's description of the process. "I remember being told I had diabetes . . . feeling out of control, different, and alone. I was only 10, and I had no sense of what diabetes was when Dr. Rich said the word to me for the first time. My parents and I had no idea how much work it would be. After I hit puberty, I started to gain a lot of weight and I felt terrible about myself . . . I thought I was fat and ugly.

When high school started, my parents backed off. I ended up doing all of my diabetes stuff myself. I guess that's how the problem began. I hated my diabetes, and I hated my weight. I tried to stop eating, but I just couldn't make myself starve. Then I figured out about the insulin. The more often I kept my sugars high, the more weight I would lose. At first, it felt great . . . I was taking control . . . eating whatever I wanted and skipping insulin. But the longer it went on and the more I had to lie to my parents to hide it, the more ashamed I felt. I gradually started to feel out of control . . . it ended up taking control of *me*."

IDENTIFY WHEN AN EATING DISORDER MAY BE COMPLICATING DIABETES

Recognize the Symptoms of Eating Disorders in Diabetes

Women with eating disorders and type 1 diabetes typically struggle with symptoms similar to those of eating disordered women without diabetes; however, they also have a unique symptom of caloric purging in the form of insulin omission and/or dose reduction. As such, clinicians working with adolescent and adult women with diabetes should be alert to extreme concerns about weight and body shape, unusual patterns of intense exercise (sometimes associated with frequent hypoglycemia), unusually low-calorie meal plans, unexplained elevations in A1C values, repeated problems with DKA, and amenorrhea.

Women with type 1 diabetes may use insulin manipulation (i.e., administering reduced insulin doses or omitting necessary doses altogether) as a means of caloric purging. Intentionally induced glycosuria is a powerful weight loss behavior unique to patients with type 1 diabetes. It may be that insulin manipulation or omission becomes a more significant problem as parental supervision of insulin administration decreases in late adolescence and then the problem continues to progress

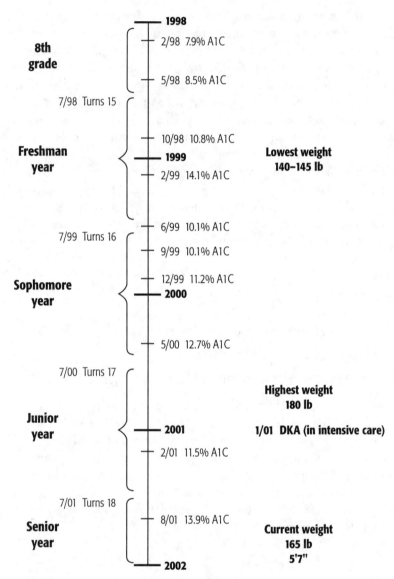

FIGURE 23.1 Timeline for case example.

throughout early adulthood (see Chapters 13 and 15). Once established as a long-standing pattern, frequent and habitual insulin omission may be a particularly difficult behavior to treat. For this reason, early detection and intervention are crucial.

Understand the Medical Risks Associated with Eating Disorders in Diabetes

As mentioned previously, studies show that recurrent insulin omission places women at heightened risk for medical complications of diabetes. Women reporting strategic insulin omission have higher A1C levels, a higher risk of developing infections, more frequent episodes of DKA, more frequent hospital and emergency room visits, and higher rates of neuropathy and retinopathy than women who do not report insulin omission. A recent investigation found that disordered eating at baseline was associated with microvascular complications of diabetes 4 years later, with 86% of highly eating disordered women presenting with retinopathy compared with 43% of moderately eating disordered women and 24% of women with no reported eating disorder.

Questions to Ask When the Presence of an Eating Disorder Is Suspected

Disordered eating behaviors are often well hidden, but patients should be encouraged to discuss issues, such as their current level of satisfaction with their weight, their weight goals, and—if willing—their experiences with binge eating. Diabetes clinicians may feel reluctant to raise these issues with their patients for fear of "teaching them how" to reduce or omit insulin for weight loss. The degree to which this is a real risk is unknown; however, given the severity of medical outcomes associated with repeated strategic insulin misuse, this risk should be taken seriously. For this reason, it is important to use sensitive, open-ended questions constructed to increase the clinicians understanding of the patient's situation without the risk of unintentionally "educating" the patient about this dangerous behavior.

Open-ended questions to consider

- How do you feel about your body weight and shape?
- (Follow-up questions to the one above) How much do you currently weigh? How much would you like to weigh ideally? How often do you weigh yourself?

- How do you like your recommended meal plan? Do you ever feel like it is hard to stick to a meal plan or like you are often eating too much or too little?
- Do you ever change your insulin dose to influence your weight (increasing or decreasing the units you take)?
- How many shots does your doctor recommend that you take each day?
- (Follow-up question to the one above) How many shots do you take on a typical day?
- What has your experience been with DKA?
- How regular is your menstrual period? (If they report regular menses, ask if they take birth control pills, which would cause a regular period despite low weight and elevated blood glucose).

KNOW HOW TO HELP WHEN THE PRESENCE OF AN EATING DISORDER IS SUSPECTED

Establish a Comprehensive Treatment Team

A multidisciplinary treatment team approach is considered the standard of care for the treatment of eating disorders. This team, when designed to treat a patient with both type 1 diabetes and an eating disorder, should include an endocrinologist specializing in diabetes, a certified diabetes educator, a nutritionist with eating disorder and/or diabetes training, a psychologist or social worker to provide weekly individual therapy, and, possibly, a psychiatrist for psychopharmacological evaluation and treatment. To provide the best quality treatment, the patient should allow all members of the team to openly communicate with each other.

Finding a mental health professional who the diabetes clinician and patient can collaborate with—optimally, someone familiar with *both* diabetes and eating disorders treatment—is the place to start. However, practitioners with these qualifications are difficult to find. A mental health professional with eating disorders treatment expertise is essential. If this clinician does not also have behavioral diabetes expertise, make sure he or she is willing to consult regularly with the diabetes clinicians on the team about the diabetes specifics.

Negotiate Realistic Treatment Goals

Patients with diabetes and eating disorders require more medical support and monitoring by a multidisciplinary team than patients with diabetes alone. Early in the treatment, they may require a medical or psychiatric inpatient hospitalization until they are medically stable enough and emotionally ready to engage in treatment as outpatients. Weekly psychotherapy is strongly recommended. Also early in the treatment, monthly appointments with the endocrinologist or nurse educator on the team may be necessary, and monthly appointments with the nutritionist are recommended. Laboratory tests (especially A1C and electrolytes) and weight checks should occur at each of the medical appointments.

With regard to diabetes management, the treatment team must be willing to set very small, attainable, incremental goals that the patient feels ready to attempt to strive toward (see Chapter 6). For a person with diabetes and an eating disorder, intensive glycemic management of diabetes is not an appropriate early treatment goal. In fact, the initial focus of treatment may be as small as prevention of future episodes of DKA. As such, patients may need to be educated about the signs and symptoms of DKA as well as its seriousness. The first goal must be to establish medical safety for the patient. Gradually, the team can build toward increases in insulin doses, increases in food intake, greater flexibility in the meal plan, regularity in eating routine, and more frequent blood glucose monitoring. With the new insulin and pump therapies currently available, flexible meal and insulin programs can be tailored for patients with genuine weight problems. A collaborative relationship with the treatment team should be established, where patients feel that their eating and weight concerns are being addressed at the same time that they are striving for improved blood glucose control.

Help patients anticipate challenges for the future, and try to problem-solve some of these challenges ahead of time. For example, the first challenge that most patients face is weight gain associated with insulin restart. Patients need to be alerted to the possibility of developing insulin edema. They should be warned that they might feel fat, bloated, and uncomfortable but that it is simply temporary water retention and not the development of fatty tissue. It may also be helpful to alert patients that treating hypoglycemia can trigger a feeling of overeating and possible weight gain. To reduce this risk, educate patients about fast treatments for hypoglycemia and appropriate serving sizes for these treatments.

Well-intentioned, caring clinicians can feel frustrated by such small and slowly attained treatment goals, especially because they do not match the recommendations of the DCCT research findings. However, when working with this at-risk patient population, taking a long-term view is crucial. The more patients feel that they can control the pace of their own treatment (see Chapter 1), the more likely they are to remain engaged in treatment and progress through it toward improved overall health and quality of life.

CONCLUSION

Eating disorders in diabetes represent some of the most complex patient problems—both medically and psychologically. The cycle of negative feelings about body image, shape, and weight; chronically elevated blood glucose levels; depression, anxiety, and shame; and poor diabetes self-care and insulin omission is difficult to treat (Figure 23.2).

Given the extent of the problem among women with diabetes and the severe medical risks associated with it, further research aimed at tar-

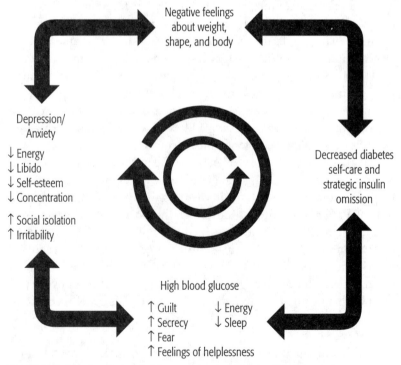

FIGURE 23.2 Model of diabetes and eating disorders/insulin omission.

geted and effective treatments is critical to the future health of this at-risk population.

ACKNOWLEDGMENTS

The author gratefully acknowledges the generous help of three terrific research assistants: Janna Fikkan, Alexa Connell, and Laura Vangsness. This work was partially funded by the Priscilla White Fellowship from the Harvard Medical School Program for Scholars in Medicine.

BIBLIOGRAPHY

Bryden KS, Neil A, Mayou RA, Peveler RC, Fairburn CG, Dunger DB: Eating habits, body weight, and insulin misuse: a longitudinal study of teenagers and young adults with type 1 diabetes. *Diabetes Care* 22:1956–1960, 1999

Carlson MG, Campbell PJ: Intensive insulin therapy and weight gain in IDDM. *Diabetes* 42:1700–1707, 1993

Fairburn CG, Peveler RC, Davies B, Mann JI, Mayou RA: Eating disorders in young adults with insulin dependent diabetes mellitus: a controlled study. *BMJ* 303:17–20, 1991

Garner DM, Garfinkel PE: *Handbook of Treatment for Eating Disorder.* 2nd ed. New York, Guilford Press, 1997

Jones JM, Lawson ML, Daneman D, Olmsted MP, Rodin G: Eating disorders in adolescent females with and without type 1 diabetes: cross sectional study. *BMJ* 320:1563–1566, 2000

Levine MD, Marcus MD: Women, diabetes, and disordered eating. *Diabetes Spectrum* 10:191–195, 1997

Polonsky WH, Anderson BJ, Lohrer PA, Aponte JE, Jacobson AM, Cole CF: Insulin omission in women with IDDM. *Diabetes Care* 17:1178–1185, 1994

Rydall AC, Rodin GM, Olmsted MP, Devenyi RG, Daneman D: Disordered eating behavior and microvascular complications in young women with insulin-dependent diabetes mellitus. *N Engl J Med* 336:1849–1854, 1997

Ann E. Goebel-Fabbri, PhD, is an Instructor in Psychiatry at Harvard Medical School and at the Behavioral and Mental Health Unit at Joslin Diabetes Center in Boston, MA.

Afterword

In closing, we would like to note several of the important themes that appear throughout the pages of this book.

First, most diabetes care is self-care, and self-care decisions are made by the person with diabetes based on that person's individual interaction style, relationships with diabetes care providers, coping abilities, emotional resources, needs, and personal stresses and limitations.

Second, effective diabetes care requires two kinds of skills: first, skill in managing specific diabetes self-care tasks, and second, skill in coping with the stresses of performing these tasks in the often-pressured and complex context of daily life.

Third, developmental, family, and cultural issues affect patients' diabetes management choices. And clinicians' understanding of these issues can often help optimize patient self-care.

Fourth, emotional distress powerfully undermines self-care, and effectively treating this distress can improve well-being and glycemic control. In many instances, the services of a mental health professional who knows about diabetes can be invaluable.

Finally, all members of the health care team should be involved in the psychological support of patients and their families. Clinicians who find ways to do this effectively will see their patients' outcomes improve and their own job satisfaction rise.

We hope that this book accomplishes the goal we set in creating it: to translate the latest psychological knowledge in diabetes into useful information for clinicians.

Barbara J. Anderson, PhD
Richard R. Rubin, PhD, CDE

Index

About the American Diabetes Association

The American Diabetes Association is the nation's leading voluntary health organization supporting diabetes research, information, and advocacy. Its mission is to prevent and cure diabetes and to improve the lives of all people affected by diabetes. The American Diabetes Association is the leading publisher of comprehensive diabetes information. Its huge library of practical and authoritative books for people with diabetes covers every aspect of self-care—cooking and nutrition, fitness, weight control, medications, complications, emotional issues, and general self-care.

To order American Diabetes Association books: Call 1-800-232-6733. Or log on to http://store.diabetes.org

To join the American Diabetes Association: Call 1-800-806-7801. www.diabetes.org/membership

For more information about diabetes or ADA programs and services: Call 1-800-342-2383. E-mail: Customerservice@diabetes.org or log on to www.diabetes.org

To locate an ADA/NCQA Recognized Provider of quality diabetes care in your area: www.ncqa.org/dprp/

To find an ADA Recognized Education Program in your area: Call 1-888-232-0822. www.diabetes.org/recognition/education.asp

To join the fight to increase funding for diabetes research, end discrimination, and improve insurance coverage: Call 1-800-342-2383. www.diabetes.org/advocacy

To find out how you can get involved with the programs in your community: Call 1-800-342-2383. See below for program Web addresses.

- *American Diabetes Month:* Educational activities aimed at those diagnosed with diabetes—month of November. www.diabetes.org/ADM
- *American Diabetes Alert:* Annual public awareness campaign to find the undiagnosed—held the fourth Tuesday in March. www.diabetes.org/alert
- *The Diabetes Assistance & Resources Program (DAR):* diabetes awareness program targeted to the Latino community. www.diabetes.org/DAR
- *African American Program:* diabetes awareness program targeted to the African American community. www.diabetes.org/africanamerican
- *Awakening the Spirit: Pathways to Diabetes Prevention & Control:* diabetes awareness program targeted to the Native American community. www.diabetes.org/awakening

To find out about an important research project regarding type 2 diabetes: www.diabetes.org/ada/research.asp

To obtain information on making a planned gift or charitable bequest: Call 1-888-700-7029. www.diabetes.org/ada/plan.asp

To make a donation or memorial contribution: Call 1-800-342-2383. www.diabetes.org/ada/cont.asp